ORIGINAL THINKERS™

-TRAILBLAZERS IN -

MEDICINE

SUSAN ALDRIDGE

This edition published in 2015 by:
The Rosen Publishing Group, Inc.
29 East 21st Street
New York, NY 10010

Additional end matter copyright © 2015 by The Rosen
Publishing Group, Inc.

Library of Congress Cataloging-in-Publication Data

Aldridge, Susan.
Trailblazers in medicine / Susan Aldridge.
    pages cm. — (Original thinkers)
Includes bibliographical references and index.
Audience: 8-12
ISBN 978-1-4777-8150-0 (library bound)
1. Physicians—Biography. 2. Medical scientists—Biography.
3. Medical innovations—History. 4. Medicine—History. I.
Title.
R134.A46 2015
610.92'2—dc23
                                                2014023964

Manufactured in the United States of America

© 2015 ELWIN STREET PRODUCTIONS www.elwinstreet.com

Cover Credits: Marie Curie © Hulton Archive/Getty Images; background ©
Sergey Nivens/Shutterstock.com

ORIGINAL THINKERS™

– TRAILBLAZERS IN –
MEDICINE

SUSAN ALDRIDGE

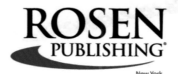

ROSEN
PUBLISHING®

New York

Contents

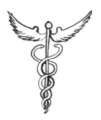

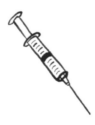

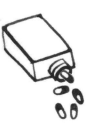

Pharmacologists

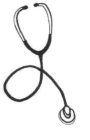

Practitioners

Introduction

Medicine has long been considered the most noble of human professions. Years before we understood the intricate and complex workings of our cells, tissues, and organs, there were men and women who sought to heal the sick and ease their suffering. This book presents the life and work of 50 individuals who have shaped the history of medicine.

Profiles of the great figures of ancient medicine, such as Galen, Hippocrates, and Avicenna, show how their knowledge laid the foundations of our modern understanding of health and disease. Their writings describe herbal remedies and surgical techniques that have inspired other doctors and led to further discoveries about the human body and how it works, in sickness and in health.

Medicine has made its greatest advances through the use of the scientific method, such as William Harvey's landmark discovery of the circulation of the blood in the early seventeenth century. Later, Louis Pasteur and Robert Koch brought about a revolution in our understanding of disease with their development of germ theory and discovery of some of the most important agents of infectious disease, such as the cholera microbe. William Withering's pioneering work on digitalis and Alexander Fleming's discovery of penicillin saved the lives of millions, and their legacies continue to form the mainstay of much medical treatment. Today we have effective medicines for diseases, including cancer, heart attack, and stroke, that would previously have been a death sentence.

Surgery was once a desperate last resort; if patients did not die of the operation, infection afterward was likely to kill them. The introduction of anesthesia allowed surgery to begin to reach its potential, while the achievements of twentieth century surgeons like Alfred Blalock heralded the modern era of cardiac surgery. Other medical advances—such as Carl Djerassi's development of the contraceptive Pill and Patrick Steptoe and Robert Edwards' work on in-vitro fertilization—have affected millions in different ways.

Above all, medicine is about compassion and care for the patient. This book would not be complete without the stories of those great men and women—Florence Nightingale, Thomas Sydenham and William Osler—whose teachings and writings have inspired doctors and nurses all over the world.

In addition to these major figures, feature sections give an overview of 10 major issues in contemporary medicine. Today's concerns are ethical, scientific, and personal. So this book looks at why medical research is still involved in animal experiments and the potential of stem cells. The genetics revolution is covered, as is the basic science of the cell, the threat of a global pandemic, and the latest advances in organ transplantation. Finally, because patient choice in healthcare is at the heart of medicine, there are features on homeopathy and herbalism—alternative medicine practices used by millions of patients—and the increasingly important topic of palliative care.

Today we face enormous medical challenges, such as the threat of pandemics, the needs of an aging population, the toll of HIV/AIDS, and major diseases for which there are still no cures. Yet we also know more than ever about how to tackle these problems and we have the weapons to do so, from vaccines and drugs to surgical procedures and patient care. All this is thanks to the dedication, knowledge, and skill of the great doctors and medical scientists of the past. Selecting only 50 figures from this elite group has been difficult, and there are many others whose contributions ought to be celebrated. But it is unquestionably true that each remarkable individual profiled here has helped to lay the foundations of twenty-first century medicine.

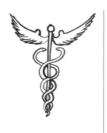

Imhotep

The ancient Egyptian polymath and god Imhotep was referred to by the great 19th-century Canadian physician Sir William Osler as "the first figure of a physician to stand out clearly from the mists of antiquity."

Born: 2650 B.C.E., Memphis, Egypt
Importance: architect and sage; first named physician in history, credited with founding medical science in Egypt
Died: 2600 B.C.E., Memphis, Egypt

What is known of Imhotep's life has been pieced together from the writings of others and from the inscriptions on statues of him. Thought until the late-19th century to have been a legendary figure, it has now been established that Imhotep lived during the Third Dynasty and may have been the son of an architect and builder. Having entered one of the temples serving the Egyptian gods as a high priest, it is likely that he would have been trained in astronomy and mathematics. From here, Imhotep entered the service of King Djoser, the second king of the Third Dynasty, becoming his second in command and chief political adviser—a remarkable rise for someone born a commoner. He also served as the Royal Architect, designing the Step Pyramid at Sakkara, thereby becoming the first named architect of a stone monument.

Although there is no firm evidence that he actually ever practiced as a physician, some ancient Egyptian and Greek accounts claim that Imhotep diagnosed and treated many different diseases, including gout, arthritis, and appendicitis, carried out surgery and dentistry, and treated illnesses with plant remedies. He is also credited with the original authorship of the *Edwin Smith Surgical Papyrus*, one of the oldest known medical texts, in which 48 case histories of injuries to the head and spine are described in great detail.

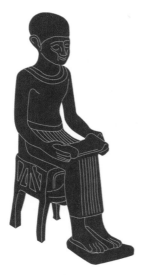

Left: Imhotep is credited with writing the earliest surviving medical text, the *Edwin Smith Surgical Papyrus*. The treatments for head and spine injuries described in the text are rational, although some magical incantations are also included.

Whatever the path of his career, it appears that Imhotep's reputation was so high that he became a god. Statues, of which many survive, show him first as an ordinary man, then as a sage bearing a papyrus, and then as a god with a beard, carrying symbols of deity. He was one of only two commoners ever to be elevated in this way, the other being the sage and healer Amenhotep, who lived several centuries later. Imhotep inspired something of a cult following, with people making pilgrimages to Egyptian temples that bore his name. Temple medicine involved various rituals and ceremonies, including incubation, where pilgrims would sleep in the temple, hoping for a healing dream in which they would come face to face with the god. Imhotep's shrines were famous both in Egypt and abroad, and many bore inscriptions from pilgrims from afar. The later Greek rulers of Egypt identified Imhotep (whom they called Imouthes) with their own healing god, Asclepius. Early Christians worshipped him too, although the cult gradually died out as Christianity spread. The great temple of Sakkara, which may have housed his tomb, was destroyed by the Roman Emperor Theodosius in 380 CE.

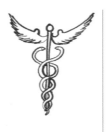

Hippocrates

The ancient Greek physician Hippocrates is perhaps best known for his *Corpus*, a body of 60 works covering many aspects of the workings of the body, its diseases and their cures. Of these works, *Aphorisms* is among the most significant, as it contains the infamous Hippocratic Oath, which proposes guidelines for a doctor's conduct toward his or her patients. The oath has had much influence on the ideal of a doctor as a compassionate, professional, dedicated, and discreet individual.

Born: 460 B.C.E., Kos, Greece
Importance: leading figure in ancient Greek medicine; his ideas on disease, healing and ethics continue to influence present-day medical practice
Died: 370 B.C.E., Thessaly, Greece

Physician and friend to the philosopher Democritus, little is known of the life of Hippocrates, although his name appears in the works of leading ancient Greek philosophers Aristotle, Socrates, Plato, and Plutarch. He may have come from a medical family, as was the tradition at the time, and seems to have taught medicine to others for a fee. He is said to have taken his cures from texts in the temple of the Greek god of medicine, Asclepius. In ancient Greece, medicine was not yet a formal discipline, and doctors were not the only people who tried to heal disease—there were also bonesetters, apothecaries, and midwives.

Hippocrates' *Corpus* is dated between 420 and 370 BCE. Unlikely to be the output of one man, the works were probably gathered together in the great library of Alexandria. They have been translated many times during the course of history, first into Latin during the sixth century, when they were introduced to Syria and the Arab world. In 1525 they were translated into Latin by Marco Fabio Calvi, and they continued to be influential as medicine developed.

The writings describe typical characteristics of ancient Greek medicine: an emphasis upon observing the patient, a willingness to debate, argue, and discuss, and a belief that diseases have a rational cause and cannot be attributed simply to divine wrath. The influence of philosophy is clear and, despite the absence of any real knowledge of human anatomy and physiology, the beginnings of a scientific approach to medicine are evident. For example, in *Airs, Waters, Places* Hippocrates discusses the role played by environmental factors in disease, describing the different illnesses found in various towns in Greece.

Hippocrates is particularly renowned for his "four-humor" theory discussed in *On the Nature of Man*, in which he suggests that health relies upon a balance between four bodily fluids: yellow bile, blood, phlegm, and black bile, and that imbalances lead to disease. In *The Sacred Disease*, he argues that epilepsy—regarded with a superstitious dread—arose from phlegm blocking the passages in the brain.

> "Help, and at least do no harm."
>
> Hippocrates

The theories of Hippocrates have influenced many other leading figures throughout the history of medicine and continue to do so today. William Harvey, who discovered the circulation of the blood (see page 24), praised Hippocrates' *On the Heart*, and the great English physician Thomas Sydenham (see page 98) was impressed by Hippocrates' observations in *Epidemics*, which comprised seven volumes of detailed case histories. Controversially, Hippocrates' writings were used in support of the practice of eugenics in Nazi Germany while, today, doctors interested in holistic treatments cite Hippocrates as the origin of their approach.

World's First Surgeon

Hua Tuo

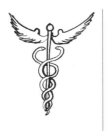

Proficient in acupuncture, gynecology, and obstetrics, ancient Chinese physician Hua Tuo is most acclaimed for his talent as a surgeon. He performed abdominal operations, such as an appendectomy to cure acute appendicitis, and what was probably the first ever colostomy to remove a diseased part of the colon. His image persists in Chinese art today and in products related to acupuncture.

Born: *c.* 110 C.E., Qiao, China
Importance: leading Chinese physician and surgeon; possibly the first to use anesthesia
Died: *c.* 207 C.E., Luoyang, China

Hua Tuo lived during the Han Dynasty, one of the great periods of Chinese history. He came from a poor family—his father died when he was seven years old—and his mother wished him to pursue a career in medicine. He studied with Dr. Cai, a close friend of his father's and also became knowledgeable in astronomy, literature, agriculture, and history.

Refusing a position in government service, Hua Tuo practiced as a physician in provinces close to his birthplace, earning a reputation as the "miracle working doctor" because he could cure his patients of their ailments with the use of just a few acupuncture points or herbal remedies. The acupuncture points on either side of the spine are named after him, as he would work on these to relieve mobility problems. Hua Tuo also developed a system of exercise called Qi Gong, which is

"The body needs exercise, but it should not be excessive. Motion consumes energy produced by food and promotes blood circulation so that the body will be free of diseases, just as a door hinge is never worm-eaten."

Hua Tuo

based upon the natural movements of five animals (tiger, deer, monkey, bear, and birds).

Hua Tuo's operations are described in the *Chronicle of the Three Kingdoms* (*c.* 270 CE) and *The Annals of the Later Han Dynasty* (430 CE). He would open up the abdomen, remove the diseased part, clean the abdominal cavity, sew up the incision, then apply a herbal ointment to help heal the wound. He devised a narcotic powder, called *Mafai San*, which was administered with wine to render the patient unconscious before surgery. The prescription has not survived, but it is thought to have contained datura flower, aconite root, rhododendron flower, or jasmine root.

Acupuncture: A system of Chinese medicine involving the insertion of fine needles at specific points on the body in order to affect the flow of energy and thereby improve health.

Hua Tuo was a Taoist and did not seek out riches or fame. He had many devoted disciples and apparently wrote many books, although none of these have survived. He was thought by many to be immortal, as he lived almost to the age of 100 and appeared always to be in perfect health. Some sources suggest he became the personal physician to Cao Cao, the ruler of the state of Wei, and was executed when Cao Cao became suspicious that Hua Tuo's prescription for surgery to treat a suspected brain tumor was an attempt to assassinate the ruler. At any rate, Hua Tuo's death marked the end of an era in Chinese medicine. Surgery was not performed again in China until reintroduced by Western doctors, as it was said to be against the teachings of Confucius. And general anesthesia was not used anywhere in the world again until 1846, when William Morton introduced ether at the Massachusetts General Hospital in Boston (see page 78).

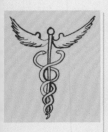

Herbalism

Humans have always found medicinal uses for plants. Some of the most important drugs in modern medicine—aspirin, morphine, and several anti-cancer drugs —were originally derived from plant sources, even if synthetic versions now prevail. The practice of "herbalism," where disease is treated using plant remedies alone, has existed for thousands of years. Today, the practice stands separate from modern Western medicine and has an important place in complementary and alternative medicine.

Plants and microbes synthesize many compounds, known as secondary metabolites, which they use to defend themselves against attack from insect pests or other microbes. These often have a biological activity that can be exploited for medicinal purposes. Toxic or brightly colored plants are often good sources of medicinal products. For example, deadly nightshade has yielded atropine and hyoscine, both of which are used in eye examination and surgery; the opium poppy has been used for its analgesic properties for at least 5,000 years, and its two active components, codeine and morphine, are still important drugs today. Meanwhile, two new antimalarial drugs—artemesin and artemether—are derived from the sweet wormwood plant, which has been used in Chinese medicine for nearly 2,000 years.

The ancient Chinese, Babylonians, Egyptians, Indians, and Native Americans all practiced herbalism. The oldest list of medicinal herbs is Shen Nung's *Pen Ts'ao*, dating back to 3000 B.C.E. The ancient Greeks and Romans also used herbal remedies, with surgeons in the Roman army spreading their knowledge throughout the Roman Empire. The Greek physicians Dioscorides and Galen (see page 16) compiled lists of herbal remedies that were subsequently in use for several hundred years. During the

Middle Ages, monasteries were an important repository of herbal knowledge in Britain and mainland Europe. The monks copied the books of Hippocrates (see page 10), Dioscorides, and Galen and grew medicinal plants in their "physick" gardens.

Elsewhere, Arabic scholars acquired herbal texts as a result of the Islamic conquest of North Africa in the seventh and eighth centuries. The Persian polymath Avicenna mentioned Greek and Roman herbal remedies in his influential *Canon of Medicine* (see page 20). With the advent of the printing press in the mid-15th century, herbal remedies were mass-produced and distributed widely. Herbalism no longer required specialist knowledge— people just used the remedies in a standardized manner, rather like today's over-the-counter equivalents.

Swiss alchemist and physician Paracelsus revived the first-century doctrine of signatures in his own practice of herbalism (see page 74). This argues that the appearance of a plant is the key to its therapeutic application, so, for example, yellow plants such as marigolds were used to cure jaundice. Astrological herbalists such as 17th-century English herbalist Nicolas Culpeper connected an affected part of the body with a specific sign and planet and prescribed the appropriate plant remedy.

During the 18th century, a split occured between traditional herbalism and the emerging sciences of botany and chemistry. The new herbalists were more interested in classifying plants and extracting and purifying their active ingredients. The first successful product of this new "grind and find" approach was digitalis, the heart drug developed by British physician William Withering in 1796 (see page 76). Withering's approach was broadly similar to that used in the pharmaceutical industry today.

In the 21st century, plants remain a treasure chest for the medicinal chemist. There are still thousands that have yet to be investigated for their medicinal properties.

Ancients

Galen of Pergamum

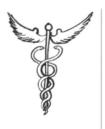

Galen was a prolific writer on physiology, diagnosis, therapy, pharmacology, and healthy living. His ideas formed the basis of the medical curriculum in Alexandria and remained largely unchallenged until the early 17th century. Possibly the most read author from this era, his books were widely translated and disseminated over the following few hundred years.

Born: 129 c.e., Pergamum, Asia Minor
Importance: Greek physician, philosopher, and writer whose ideas dominated medicine for around 1,400 years
Died: c. 216 c.e., Rome, Italy

Much of our knowledge of Galen's education and subsequent career comes from his own writings and lacks much independent historical verification. He began to study medicine at the age of 16, apparently following a dream of his father's, in which the god of healing, Asclepius, advised this. Galen's studies took him to Smyrna and Corinth and to Alexandria in Egypt, then a great center of learning. He studied for over 10 years, gaining an unusually long and varied medical education for that time.

Galen was educated in anatomy, surgery, and Hippocratic medicine and returned to Pergamum around 157 C.E. to become physician to the troupe of gladiators employed by the High Priest. In 162 C.E. he moved to Rome, where he became famous for his learning. Rome was intensely competitive, however, and Galen had many rivals. He withdrew to Pergamum for a while, returning to Rome in 169 C.E. to become physician to the Emperor Marcus Aurelius and his family. He also saw many other patients, from the high born to slaves, and people wrote to him from afar seeking medical advice.

Galen's medicine was a synthesis of the ideas of Hippocrates, Plato, and Aristotle, with a strong emphasis on rational explanation

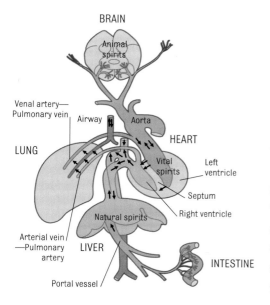

BRAIN

Animal spirits

Venal artery— Pulmonary vein

Airway

Aorta

HEART

LUNG

Vital spirits

Left ventricle

Septum

Natural spirits

Right ventricle

Arterial vein/ —Pulmonary artery

LIVER

INTESTINE

Portal vessel/

Left: Galen interpreted the circulatory system as having blood forming in the liver, flowing through the veins, and being consumed by the heart and brain. Also present in the system was "breath spirit," which consisted of animal spirits, vital spirits, and natural spirits and was fundamental to life.

and observation. He believed in Hippocrates' four humors as the basis of health (see page 10), the Platonic idea of the three main bodily systems of liver, heart, and brain being connected to mental states, and Plato's theory of the soul. He was very clear that the brain was the seat of perception and voluntary motion. Galen also wrote about the "breath spirit" or *pneuma*, which he believed flowed through the arteries, while the veins carried the blood, manufactured in the liver. His theories on the latter were not challenged until William Harvey's work on the circulation of the blood in the 1620s (see page 24).

In his practice, Galen relied on palpation, taking the pulse, and inspection of urine, and his treatments included a wide range of herbal and plant remedies. He also carried out experiments on nerves, the heart, lungs, and pulse, as well as carrying on dissection work that he probably learned in Alexandria, in order to better understand the anatomy of the human body and aid surgical procedures. Galen's influence was far-reaching, with many translations—including Henry VIII's *Hygienics*, which prescribed diet, exercise, rest, and hygiene for a healthy lifestyle.

al-Rāzā

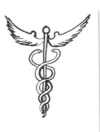

Considered to be the pioneer of pediatrics, ophthalmology, and neurosurgery, al-Rāzā believed strongly in the rational approach, experimental medicine, and the powers of observation. He was the first physician to describe the symptoms of both measles and smallpox based upon clinical examination and to be able to distinguish between them in an early example of differential diagnosis.

Born:*c.* 864 C.E., Rayy, Persia
Importance: pioneering figure in the medieval Islamic world, producing over 200 works on medicine, pharmacy, and other sciences
Died: *c.* 925 C.E., Rayy, Persia

Muhammed Ibn Zakariya al-Rāzā, known in Europe as Rhazes, worked as a physician in his home city of Rayy, near what is now Tehran, in Iran. He started his career as an alchemist, turning to medicine when the chemicals he used in his experiments apparently affected his eyes. He was also knowledgeable about music and philosophy. Widely traveled, he served at the Samanid Court of Central Asia, in both his native city and in Baghdad.

Of lasting significance, al-Rāzā's *Book on Smallpox and Measles* was translated from Arabic into Latin in the 18th century and was influential in the early days of inoculation against smallpox. Between 1498 and 1866 it was published in 40 different editions in Europe and translated into various languages. In the book, al-Rāzā observes that "thin, hot, and dry" bodies are more likely to get measles than smallpox while "thin, cold, and dry" bodies are unlikely to get either disease, but if they get smallpox it will be only mild. Elsewhere in the book, al-Rāzā describes the symptoms of both diseases in detail, carefully explaining which are common and which specific to either disease. Other chapters deal with the prevention and treatment of smallpox and the prognosis for both diseases. The book is considered a landmark in the history of medicine, for smallpox has killed millions of people over the course of human history (see also Edward Jenner, page 46). It was not until 1979 that science overcame smallpox, through vaccination, and eradicated it worldwide (the last recorded case was in 1978). Although al-Rāzā lived and worked long before the germ theory of disease was established (see page 60), his book does mention "putrefying air" as a contributory factor in the spread of smallpox.

Prognosis: A medical opinion, based upon signs and symptoms, on the likely course and outcome of a disease.

Another famous publication, the *Comprehensive Book of Medicine*, contained extracts from previous medical authors alongside detailed case histories from his own practice. In this, al-Rāzā sometimes criticized Galen's ideas (see page 16), challenging the courses laid down by him. This work was translated into Latin in 1279 by Faraj ben Salim, a physician of Sicilian-Jewish origin, employed by King Charles of Anjou to translate medical texts. Running to 23 volumes, it is an important source of Greek, Indian and early Arabic writings on medicine, since al-Rāzā was meticulous about recording his sources.

His most influential work in Europe was a shorter general medical text called *Book of Medicine Dedicated to Mansur* (the Governor of Rayy) written *c.* 903 C.E. Many editions were produced during the Renaissance era with commentary by leading physicians of the day, such as Vesalius (see page 22). In addition to this, al-Rāzā also wrote about pediatrics, the bladder, and the kidneys and was the first to link hay fever to exposure to roses. His medical texts were used as teaching aids throughout the Middle East and Europe, up to the 18th century.

Avicenna

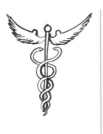

Avicenna developed a system of medicine that is famous for synthesizing elements of Eastern and Western knowledge—including Galen's work—Islamic medicine, Aristotelian philosophy, and some ideas from traditional Indian medicine. A national hero in Iran, Avicenna is revered as one of the greatest Persians who ever lived.

Born: 980, Afshana, Central Asia

Importance: leading Islamic physician and philosopher whose writings influenced medical education for several hundred years

Died: 1037, Hamedan, Central Asia

Avicenna is the European name of Ibn Sina, who lived in the so-called Golden Age of Islam (*c.* 700–1200), when knowledge of mathematics, philosophy, and medicine blossomed. Avicenna was a child prodigy—he mastered mathematics, science, and philosophy at a young age and began his study of medicine at the age of 16. By 18, he was already a practicing physician and attended the Samani ruler Nuh ibn Mansur, who allowed him to use the royal library to extend his knowledge. Following the death of his father, Avicenna traveled widely, acting on occasions as vizier to local leaders or emirs. At the same time, he busied himself with teaching and writing.

> "Medicine is not one of the difficult sciences, and therefore, I excelled in it in a very short time."
>
> Avicenna

A profilic writer, Avicenna is credited with having produced as many as 450 works, of which 240 survive. Of these, 40 concern medicine while others are on music, geometry, astronomy, religion, and philosophy. His most noted medical work is his 14-volume *Canon of Medicine*, which was translated into Latin by Gerard of Cremona in the 12th century and subsequently introduced into

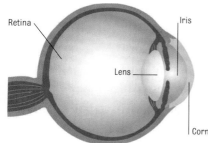

Left: Avicenna was the first person to correctly describe the anatomy of the human eye, as well as the physiology of eye movements. These went on to form the basis of modern ophthalmology.

Retina

Iris

Lens

Cornea

Europe. The *Canon* consists of five different books and one million words covering general principles; pharmacology; diseases specific to a given organ; non-specific diseases, like fever; and recipes for remedies. The pharmacology work lists 760 drugs with comments on their effectiveness.

The Arabic text of the *Canon* was printed in Rome in 1593, making it one of the first Arabic texts in print. Owing to its encyclopedic content and its structured layout, it soon replaced the works of Galen and al-Rāzā (see pages 16 and 18) in its importance to the growing medical profession and remained a key volume up until the 18th century. The *Canon* continued as a medical text in the Islamic world long after it had been superseded in Europe and is still valued today in certain medical schools in India and Pakistan.

Avicenna introduced many medical concepts that are still familiar today, such as risk factors; the importance of diet, climate, and environment in health; clinical trials; contagion; quarantine; and experimental medicine. He was the first to describe the anatomy of the human eye and eye diseases such as cataract. He also realized that tuberculosis was contagious and that diseases can be spread through soil and water. Furthermore, Avicenna was the first to take a clinical interest in psychology and psychiatry and is credited, through his interest in chemistry, as an early pioneer of aromatherapy.

Andreas Vesalius

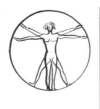

With a deep-rooted conviction that knowledge of anatomy was essential for successful surgery, Andreas Vesalius produced a milestone in medical science when he published *On the Structure of the Human Body* in 1543. Based on research using human dissection, the book gave precise descriptions and illustrations of the human skeleton, muscles, nervous system, blood vessels, and organs. Controversial at the time of publication, the work challenged Galen's theories on anatomy, which had dominated for well over a thousand years (see page 16).

Born: 1514, Brussels, Belgium

Importance: leading figure in Renaissance medicine, who used human dissection studies to lay the groundwork for modern anatomy

Died: 1564, Zakynthos, Greece

The son of a Brussels pharmacist, Vesalius began his study of medicine at Louvain in Belgium in 1528, moving to Paris in 1533. He returned to Louvain in 1536, as a result of war in France, and subsequently studied in Padua. It was common for doctors to study in several cities in this way during the Renaissance period, gathering information from the leading centers of knowledge. After a short period as a military surgeon, he took up a professorship in anatomy and surgery at the University of Padua at the age of 24.

Vesalius became famous for carrying out human dissections himself, rather than leaving the work to an assistant, and used this as a tool for research into human anatomy. Until this time, dissection had been used mainly for instruction (even this was controversial, as it went against many religious traditions to cut into the human body). His interest increased when a Paduan judge became fascinated by his work and allowed him to work with the bodies of executed criminals. The outcome, *On the Structure of the Human Body*, was one of the first collaborations between an anatomist and an artist trained in anatomy. The woodcut illustrations—probably produced by German artist Jan van Calcar—represent the dissected human body in naturalistic poses. Through his human dissection studies, Vesalius discovered new structures such as the thalamus.

Crucially, Vesalius criticized Galen's medicine, which had until this time held sway in the medical profession. Galen based his anatomy upon the dissection of Barbary apes, rather than humans, and the anatomy of the two differ in important ways. For example, Vesalius challenged Galen's claim that there is a passage between the two ventricles of the heart through which blood can pass.

Thalamus: Part of the lower brain that relays nerve impulses carrying sensory information from the spinal cord to the cerebral cortex.

Vesalius's work was highly controversial and met with considerable resistance in Padua and, subsequently, in Spain, where he became physician to King Charles V and then, in 1555, to his son, Philip II. However, the tide of opinion began to turn and, by the end of the 16th century, the view of human anatomy presented by Vesalius had become the "gold standard" in medicine and was widely translated and disseminated.

Vesalius's work laid foundations for more detailed studies of human organs by physicians such as the Italian anatomist Marcello Malpighi, who published important works on the structure of the lungs, skin, liver, and brain (see also Giovanni Battista Morgagni, page 26). Vesalius's accurate understanding of human anatomy was also essential to William Harvey's work on the circulation of the blood (see page 24) and to other work promoting the view of the human body as an efficient machine.

William Harvey

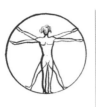

In 1628, William Harvey published *On the Motions of the Heart and Blood*, which discussed his ideas on circulation. The work met with resistance in Europe, as it challenged Galen's theories on the manufacture of blood, which had held sway for over a thousand years. In Britain, however, the work was received with great enthusiasm and has since become a scientific classic, marking the start of our modern understanding of physiology.

Born: 1578, Folkestone, England
Importance: discovered the circulation of the blood and so founded modern physiology
Died: 1657, London, England

Harvey attended school in Canterbury and studied medicine at Cambridge University. On graduating, in 1597, he went to Padua, the leading medical school, for further studies. Among Harvey's teachers at Padua was anatomist Girolamo Fabrizio, who discovered the valves in veins, publishing his findings in 1603. Fabrizio could not explain the function of these valves, however, and it was this puzzle that triggered Harvey's interest in how blood traveled through the body. He soon had a clear idea of some kind of circulatory system, stating that: "The movement of the blood occurs constantly in a circulatory manner and is the result of the beating of the heart."

Returning to London in 1602, Harvey established himself as a physician. He became a Fellow of the Royal College of Physicians in 1607, and obtained a position as physician at St. Bartholomew's Hospital in 1609. Beginning in 1618, he attended King James I and, later, his son, King Charles I. Alongside his medical practice, he continued to carry out animal dissections and experiments in pursuit of his ideas on circulation. He first presented his work to the Royal College of Physicians in 1616.

In *On the Motions of the Heart and Blood*, also known as *De*

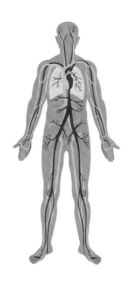

Left: William Harvey was the first person to accurately describe the circulatory system, showing how blood originates in the heart, before flowing to all parts of the body through the arteries, then being brought back to the heart through the veins.

Motu Cordis, he discussed his theory on the working of the heart and circulation. It described how valves in the heart, veins, and arteries allowed for a one-way movement of the blood. With the heart acting as a muscular pump, it contracted to expel blood into the arteries, which carried it to the organs. The right ventricle (lower chamber) of the heart supplied the lungs, where blood was oxygenated, while the left ventricle supplied blood to the rest of the body. Blood then flowed back to the heart through the veins. Such a proposal directly challenged Galen's long-accepted theory that blood was made in the liver and flowed to the organs, whereupon it was consumed (see page 16). Nevertheless, a number of young English researchers carried out further experiments on blood circulation and Harvey's theories soon superseded those of Galen.

William Harvey also worked on reproduction and was the first to suggest that humans, and other mammals, reproduced by the fertilization of an egg by sperm—this came two centuries before mammalian eggs were actually discovered. In 1651, he published *On the Generation of Animals,* which was well received. He also carried out research on animal locomotion, which remained undiscovered until 1959.

The Body

Giovanni Battista Morgagni

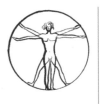

Giovanni Battista Morgagni was a firm believer that diagnosis could be based upon the study of the human cadaver. He argued that the symptoms, and causes, of a disease would reveal themselves in pathological lesions apparent after death. He was therefore the first to propose that disease was located in specific organs. His ideas were an extension of the rational approach to medicine proposed by the great anatomist Marcello Malpighi (1628–1694).

Born: 1682, Forli, Italy
Importance: founder of organ pathology through studies linking postmortem findings to the cause and symptoms of disease
Died: 1771, Padua, Italy

Morgagni studied at the University of Bologna from 1698 to 1707. He was taught by the followers of Malpighi and eventually became personal assistant to one of them, Antonio Valsava. Having gained his degree in philosophy and medicine in 1701, Morgagni sought further experience in anatomy at leading hospitals in Bologna. He kept a detailed medical and scientific journal from 1699 to 1767, in which he recorded case histories, lecture notes and postmortem findings.

Marcello Malpighi's work had marked the beginning of so-called rational medicine, rooted in anatomy. It was still controversial, and when Morgagni took up the Malpighian crusade in Bologna, he made a number of enemies. Moving to Venice in 1707, he studied chemistry and carried out a number of postmortem examinations with Gian Domenico Santorini, a lecturer in anatomy at the Venetian Medical College. Morgagni returned to his hometown of Forli for a while, before becoming professor of medicine at the great medical school of Padua in 1711; a Chair of Anatomy was created for him there, in 1715, and he remained at Padua until his death.

Morgagni's international reputation was established in 1706, when he published his *Notes on Anatomy*, which records many of his key research studies on fine anatomy. He discovered many new anatomical structures in the human body—in the male and female genital organs, for example, and in the trachea, or windpipe. Several of these are named after him, such as Morgagni's columns in the rectum and Morgagni's pyramid in the thyroid gland. Morgagni also described many diseases for the first time, thanks to his anatomical studies, including tuberculosis of the kidney and cirrhosis of the liver.

In 1761, Morgagni published *On the Sites and Causes of Diseases*, which was the culmination of his life's work and contained the material from his years of journals. The work focuses on Malpighi's idea that the body is a complex machine, subject to breakdown and wear. Morgagni argued that the resulting lesions would reveal themselves in the body's anatomical structures. The work consists of five volumes covering the brain; the heart and lungs; the digestive and reproductive systems; fevers; tumors; and miscellaneous diseases. This medical classic contains 700 case histories, most of them Morgagni's own work, but also some of Valsava's posthumous cases. Morgagni also carried out a comprehensive revision of existing medical literature, comparing the observations of others with his own. The volume was soon translated into English, German, and French, and became required reading for students in the leading medical schools of the day, including Leiden and Vienna.

Morgagni became a great inspiration to others. The Scottish anatomist Matthew Baillie continued to identify and classify organic lesions, while René Théophile Hyacinthe Laënnec, the inventor of the stethoscope (see page 48), looked for pathological lesions in living subjects, and Rudolf Virchow used advances in microscopy to take pathology from the level of the organ to the level of the individual cells that make up the organ (see page 32).

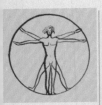

The Cell

The cell is the basic building block of life. It is a tiny compartment that separates all the components and compounds important for sustaining life from the outer environment. Bacteria, the simplest organisms, consist of just a single cell, while the human body contains around 50 million million cells. A cell cannot be seen with the naked eye, and it was not until the invention of the microscope that cells could be studied. They were first described by the English scientist and inventor Robert Hooke in the 1660s.

In 1838, German botanist Matthias Schleiden suggested that all plant tissues are made out of cells. The following year his associate Theodor Schwann went further by suggesting that all life is made of cells. Despite this, biologists were still not sure where cells came from. One popular idea was that of "spontaneous generation," suggesting that cells were suddenly created, apparently out of nothing. This theory was disproved by Rudolf Virchow and Louis Pasteur, however, who established one of the major tenets of cell theory—that cells come from other cells, by dividing into two (see pages 32 and 54).

A bacterial cell is about one micrometer in diameter, while an animal cell is some 10 to 30 micrometers in diameter. Plant cells are bigger, ranging from 10 to 100 micrometers in diameter. In complex organisms, cells join together to form tissues, like blood or muscle, and these in turn form structures known as organs, like skin or the heart, which are generally composed of more than one kind of tissue. There are about 200 different cell types in the body, each with different characteristics and functions. Therefore, a red blood cell carries oxygen, while a neuron sends and receives electrochemical signals, thereby communicating information between brain and body.

With the exception of neurons, which generally last for the whole lifetime of the body, most cells have a limited lifetime. The cells lining the stomach are renewed every two days, while a liver cell has a lifetime of 18 months. All cells come from primitive cells called "stem cells" by a process known as differentiation (see Stem Cells and Cloning, page 64).

Increasingly sophisticated microscopic techniques, developed since the 19th century, have revealed that the cell contains many different structures called organelles, floating in a watery fluid called cytoplasm. The nucleus of the cell contains deoxyribonucleic acid (DNA), the chemical genes are made of, combined with protein molecules, in tiny threadlike structures called chromosomes.

Enzyme: A molecule which catalyzes (speeds up) biochemical reactions in cells, such as the breakdown of glucose to release energy.

Genes are transcribed into messenger ribonucleic acid (RNA) within the nucleus, where it is translated into protein molecules in organelles called ribosomes. These proteins are mainly enzymes. Other organelles, such as the endoplasmic reticulum, the Golgi apparatus, and lysosomes, are involved in the processing, transportation, and breakdown of protein molecules respectively. The cell is enclosed by a membrane made up of a double layer of lipid molecules, allowing materials to go in and out of the cell.

Like all complex machines, the cell sometimes goes wrong. Disease is now understood increasingly in cellular, molecular, and genetic terms. Thus, one new theory about cancer is that it results from a defect in apoptosis, the suicide of damaged cells, when the genes controlling this process are damaged. Defective cells are allowed to survive and therefore may start to form a tumor.

The Body

Claude Bernard

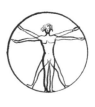

More interested in medical research than practice, Claude Bernard believed that physiology, pathology, and pharmacology were closely linked and that all three should be considered as sciences on a par with physics and chemistry. He challenged the long-held view that the body was a collection of autonomous organs at the mercy of its outer environment. Instead, he proposed what he called the "internal milieu" of the body, according to which the body creates its own inner environment where fluids, cells, and organs work in equilibrium with one another in health, while illness disrupts the balance.

Born: 1813, St. Julien de Villefranche, France
Importance: pioneer of experimental physiology, making key discoveries in digestion, the nervous system, and toxicology
Died: 1878, Paris, France

Bernard studied medicine in Paris, qualifying in 1839. Tutored by François Magendie, a leading researcher in physiology who was also involved in animal research, Bernard later became his research assistant at the Collège de France. Bernard had great manual dexterity and an approach to the design of his experiments that was firmly based upon scientific theory. He developed many new techniques and approaches in animal experimentation.

"The true worth of an experimenter consists in his pursuing not only what he seeks in his experiment, but also what he did not seek."

Claude Bernard

One of Bernard's major discoveries, in 1848, showed the role of the pancreas in digestion. He demonstrated, from his experiments, that the pancreas secreted enzymes that break down fat, protein, and carbohydrates. For this work, he received an award for experimental physiology from the French Academy of Sciences.

Other experiments on the digestive system showed the presence of an enzyme in the gastric juices of the stomach and the alteration of carbohydrates into simple sugars before absorption in the gastrointestinal tract. He also found that the liver stored glucose from food, as glycogen, and was able to release it as needed to keep blood-glucose levels steady. Bernard also carried out important work on toxicology, studying the poison "curare," used as a weapon by South American Indians. Curare acts where the nerve meets the muscle, stopping the nerve from contracting the muscle, so causing widespread paralysis. He also studied the mode of action of carbon monoxide and opium. Bernard was able to show that the action of poisons and drugs are specific to targets within the body. Through animal experiments carried out in 1852 to 1853, he also showed the vasomotor effect of nerves, where they can either contract or dilate the blood vessels, so playing an important role in regulating the temperature of the body. He also studied fetal physiology and the role of the placenta. Bernard's great work *Introduction to the Study of Experimental Medicine* was published in 1865.

Glucose: A simple sugar used as the body's basic fuel and derived from the carbohydrates in the diet.

In 1852, Magendie retired and Bernard took over most of his work at the Collège de France. In 1854, a professorship of general physiology was created for him at the Sorbonne. When Magendie died, Bernard succeeded him as Professor of Medicine. Bernard received much recognition for his work during his lifetime. He gained an Academy of Sciences award for his work on the nervous system, was elected a member of the Academie Française, and became President of the French Academy. When he died in 1878, he was given a public funeral, becoming the first-ever French scientist to receive this honor.

Rudolf Virchow

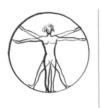

Suspicious of the "germ theory" put forward by his contemporary Louis Pasteur (see pages 54 and 60), Rudolf Virchow believed that disease came from within the body and not from external, infectious agents. In 1858, he published a book on cellular pathology in which he claimed that the cell was the basic unit of life, capable of reproducing itself. A radical view for its time, going against the popular view that life somehow arose spontaneously, this idea was nevertheless soon supported by Pasteur's experiments on microbes.

Born: 1821, Schivelbein, Pomerania (now Germany)
Importance: placed the cell at the center of the understanding of disease and founded the science of cellular pathology
Died: 1902, Berlin, Germany

Virchow studied medicine in Berlin, graduating in 1842, and gained a junior position at the city's leading hospital, the Charité. However, he lost his job in 1848, owing to his liberal political views. He subsequently moved to the city of Würzburg, where he became Professor of Pathological Anatomy. In 1856, he returned to Berlin to take up a position created for him at the newly established pathology institute at the university there. Virchow was also involved in the Franco-German war, when he led the first hospital train to the front line to help wounded soldiers.

Using developments in microscopy—such as the development of stains for tissues and cells, and the microtome, which cuts very thin slices of tissue for study—Virchow promoted the use of the microscope to advance the study of pathology and make major discoveries. He described leukemia, a group of blood cancers, in 1845, and was also one of the first to study inflammation, embolism, and thrombosis (the last two being abnormal formations of blood clots) at the cellular level. He was the first to put forward the idea that a venous thrombosis in the leg could

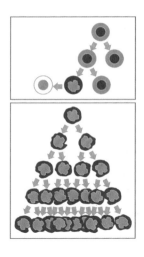

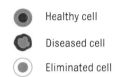

Healthy cell

Diseased cell

Eliminated cell

Left: Virchow's work on the cellular basis of disease showed that while damaged cells are normally eliminated by the body in a process called apoptosis (top), cancerous cells can evade this system and multiply freely (bottom).

break off and travel to the lung, forming a potentially fatal embolism. In 1874 Virchow introduced the first standard procedure for conducting an autopsy that is still used today.

Virchow was greatly influenced by the work of Mathias Schleiden (1804–1881) and Theodore Schwann (1810–1882), German biologists working on the importance of the cell in biology and medicine. Schleiden claimed that plants were made up of cells, while Schwann had discovered that cells were the basic building blocks of all the animal tissues he studied. Their research led Virchow to believe that disease began in the cells. He argued that disease and its symptoms either resulted from an abnormality within the cells, or from cells' response to some kind of stimulus. His work revealed the cellular basis of cancer, which is still the basis of modern views of the disease, where one abnormal cell multiplies to form a tumor.

Virchow was a man of many interests. He was involved in anthropology and archeology, working on excavations hoping to uncover the ancient Greek city of Troy. He also believed that a doctor could be a vehicle for social reform. He was influential in improving public health in Germany: As a member of Berlin City Council, he advised on a number of issues, including sewage disposal, school hygiene, and the inspection of meat.

The Body

Henry Gray

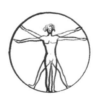

Henry Gray's name is synonymous with the textbook on human anatomy that he and his colleague in surgery created for their students in the mid-19th century. Conceived in 1855, *Gray's Anatomy: Descriptive and Surgical* was first published in 1858.

Updated and revised in keeping with advances in our knowledge and understanding of anatomy, the book remains the "doctor's bible" to this day.

Born: 1827, Windsor, England
Importance: author of *Gray's Anatomy: Descriptive and Surgical*, the world's most famous medical text
Died: 1861, London, England

Little is known of Gray's childhood and schooling, but he enrolled as a medical student in St. George's Hospital in south London at the age of 18. He became a demonstrator and lecturer in human anatomy, peforming many dissections himself, and also worked as a surgeon. He was elected as a Fellow of the Royal Society at the early age of 25 and, a year later, won the prestigious Astley Cooper award for his research on the structure and function of the spleen.

When Gray and his colleague Dr. Henry Vandyke Carter decided to produce their textbook, they spent 18 months working together on dissections in order to gather the necessary material. Carter was a superb draftsman and created a series of woodcut illustrations, while Gray composed the accompanying text. The result was a 750-page volume with 363 illustrations. It was the quality of Carter's illustrations—large, clear and functional, with the labels incorporated within the images—that set this apart from other texts in anatomy, which tended to be pocket sized. Some of Carter's images were even life-size, which was a remarkable aid to learning.

The book came to be known simply as *Gray's Anatomy* and, over the years, many editions have been produced in the

United Kingdom and the United States. Color was first introduced into the illustrations in 1887, when the 11th edition was published. Although it no longer contains any of its original text or illustrations, the concept has endured and the book remains an important resource for medical students, medical professionals, and medical illustrators. The 39th edition runs to 1,600 pages, has 2,260 illustrations, and weighs about 11 pounds. Its editor, Professor Susan Standring of King's College London, has revised the text according to body regions, rather than systems—the original arrangement—as this is more in keeping with the way modern clinicians work. The work is also available online and is said to be the world's largest single source of anatomical information.

Henry Gray would likely have achieved much in his medical career. However, he died of smallpox at the age of 34, while caring for a nephew who had the disease. Carter, who left for India and a career in tropical medicine before the book was published, died in 1897.

The status, and practice, of anatomy has changed since Gray's time. Once a discipline in its own right, it is now part of mainstream medicine and dentistry, along with the study of physiology. Anatomy can be defined as the study of the structures of the body—such as bones, nerves, muscles, organs, and so on. It now encompasses histology, the study of tissue, and cytology, the study of cells themselves. Dissection of the body is no longer used routinely in medical education, although it is still essential for carrying out a postmortem. Visual aids and computer techniques have taken the place of dissection, but *Gray's Anatomy* remains an important teaching aid.

Wilhelm Konrad Röntgen

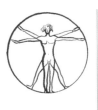

Recipient of the first-ever Nobel Prize for Physics, in 1901, physicist Wilhelm Röntgen made a remarkable discovery that will always be associated with his name—the X-ray. One of the most significant developments in the history of medicine, the X-ray eliminated the need for surgery in order to see inside the body. Used widely since the turn of the twentieth century, it remains the most commonly used medical diagnostic test to this day.

Born: 1845, Lennep, Germany
Importance: discovered X-rays, one of the most important medical diagnostic tools
Died: 1923, Munich, Germany

Röntgen studied physics in the Netherlands and mechanical engineering in Zurich and then worked in various academic positions in German universities, teaching physics and carrying out research.

In 1895, while he was Professor of Physics at the University of Würzburg, Röntgen discovered X-rays. He was working with a discharge tube, in which an electric discharge passes through a glass tube at low pressure. Röntgen noticed as the electric discharge passed through the glass tube, a card coated with barium platinocyanide on the other side of the laboratory became fluorescent.

Röntgen had discovered a new form of radiation, which he called X-rays. He experimented further and found that the rays could darken a photographic plate. By placing pieces of card between his radiation source and the photographic plate, he saw the radiation was absorbed to a varying extent depending on the thickness of the card. Quick to see the potential of his discovery, Röntgen held the hand of his wife, Anna, over the photographic plate in the path of the X-rays. The result was the first ever X-ray, now famous, in which Anna's bones appear white, the flesh of her hand black and the ring on her finger an opaque shadow.

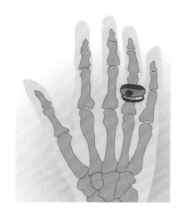

Left: Röntgen's first public demonstration of X-rays took place during a lecture in Würzburg in 1865, when he made an X-ray of the hand of respected anatomist Dr. Albert von Kölliker. The picture clearly showed the bones of Kölliker's hand, and even the ring on his finger.

Röntgen showed that X-rays were another form of electromagnetic radiation, like visible, ultraviolet, and infrared light, but of a much shorter wavelength and higher frequency. The following year, a conference of doctors in Chicago marveled at X-ray pictures showing the bones of the arm and leg of a subject. The medical applications were seized upon almost immediately.

The X-ray proved a success because body tissues absorb its rays to different extents. X-rays are focused on the body part being investigated and a photographic film is positioned close by to detect the emerging radiation. Bone absorbs X-rays well, and so appears white on the film. Soft tissue absorbs the radiation less well and appears dark, because more radiation passes through that part of the body to strike the film. Metal objects, like jewelry and pacemakers, appear as opaque shadows.

In the early days, X-rays took the guesswork out of diagnosing tuberculosis, which had previously been done by listening to chest sounds. It also allowed better assessment of limb fractures and prevented many amputations. Godfrey Hounsfield, the British physicist, developed computer-assisted tomography in the 1950s, in which X-ray images were analyzed by computer to give three-dimensional images of the human body. Known as CT scanning, this has since become an important imaging technique in its own right.

The Body

Karl Landsteiner

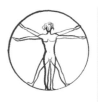

Karl Landsteiner is most famous for his work on the human blood group system, through which he determined that there were three distinct human blood groups (a fourth was discovered later). Through his analysis of these blood groups, and the way in which they react when mixed together, Landsteiner was able to establish a rule for the safe transfusion of blood from one person to another, eliminating the possibility of rejection.

Born: 1868, Vienna, Austria
Importance: discovered blood groups and so laid the foundations for safe blood transfusion
Died: 1943, New York, United States

Karl Landsteiner graduated in medicine in 1891 and went on to study chemistry in Germany and Switzerland, with some of the leading professors of the day, including the great Emil Fischer. His interest in serology (the study of blood serum) and immunology began when he took up a position at the department of hygiene at the University of Vienna in 1896. Later, he moved to the pathology department, where he carried out, or assisted at, nearly 4,000 postmortem examinations. In 1909, he was elected to the Chair of Pathology at the University of Vienna.

In 1900, Landsteiner published an important paper on the interagglutination (a type of clumping together) that sometimes took place if blood cells from one person were mixed with blood serum from someone else—a phenomenon that posed a barrier to successful blood transfusion. He carried out a series of experiments from which arose the three human blood groups— A, B, and O. A and B stand for specific protein molecules called "antigens" that are attached to the surface of A and B blood cells respectively. Cells belonging to blood group O bear neither A nor B on their surfaces, while AB blood cells carry both. Each blood sera contains molecules called "antibodies," which bind to the corresponding antigen and cause agglutination reaction. For example, group A serum contains anti-B, while group B contains anti-A; group O serum contains anti-A and anti-B antibodies, while group AB serum contains neither. Thus Landsteiner's rule was that serum contains only those antibodies that are *not* active against its own blood group. This meant that a person with AB blood could receive any blood cells, while a person with group O blood could receive only group O blood cells.

Landsteiner began to look for other differences in human blood and conducted research into syphilis and poliomyelitis (polio). In 1906, he managed to infect monkeys with syphilis and to carry out experiments with the causative agent *Spirochaeta pallida*, thereby developing the Wasserman test for diagnosis of the disease. After carrying out a postmortem on a child who died of polio, he injected an extract from the brain and spinal cord into various experimental animals and managed to reproduce the disease. He found no bacteria and concluded: "The supposition is hence near, that a so-called invisible virus or a virus belonging to the class of protozoa, causes the disease" (although we now know viruses and protozoa are completely different types of microbe).

In 1919, Landsteiner became dissatisfied with working conditions in Vienna and moved to The Hague, then the United States in 1922, taking up a position at the Rockefeller Institute and becoming an American citizen in 1929. In 1930, he received the Nobel Prize for Physiology or Medicine in recognition of his work on the ABO blood groups. Then, in 1940, Landsteiner, Alexander Wiener, and Philip Levine discovered a new factor, called Rhesus factor, in blood. A woman lacking Rhesus factor produces antibodies against a Rhesus-positive fetus, which can destroy the child's red blood cells, resulting in jaundice and brain damage. Their discovery meant that the problem could be anticipated, and affected children could then be saved by blood transfusion.

The Body

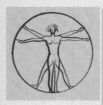

The Genetics Revolution

Advances in gene technology, such as deoxyribonucleic-acid (DNA) sequencing, led to the completion of the Human Genome Project (HGP) in 2000 (see page 44) and opened up new possibilities in diagnosing and treating disease. The HGP revealed that humans have fewer genes than was previously believed—around 30,000, instead of the expected 100,000.

Each gene codes for a protein, which plays a role in some biochemical or physiological function, such as transmitting nerve impulses or making the heart beat. Each gene is made up of a stretch of DNA carrying a chemical code specifying the molecular nature of its protein. Any aberration in the code, known as a mutation, can lead to a dysfunctional protein, which may cause disease. For example, mutations in the gene for Factor VIII, found in people with hemophilia, cause the blood to stop clotting.

Even before the HGP, genetics researchers were developing tests for so-called single gene disorders like cystic fibrosis, hemophilia, and sickle cell anemia. In such disorders, there is a simple relationship between carrying a mutated gene and developing a disease. Therefore, people with a family history of a genetic disorder can find out their chance of having an affected child. This has led to the introduction of preimplantation genetic diagnosis, a combination of in vitro fertilization (IVF) and genetic testing, in which a number of embryos are created by IVF and a single cell taken from each one for DNA analysis. Those embryos found not to carry a gene mutation are implanted into the woman's uterus. The couple can continue with the pregnancy, confident that they are carrying a healthy child. The alternative is to test the fetus during pregnancy and then make the difficult decision whether to terminate an affected fetus. Preimplantation genetic diagnosis is now available for a range of single-gene disorders such as Huntington's chorea and sickle cell anemia.

Genes have also been discovered that are linked to cancer. Around five percent of breast cancer cases occur among women with a family history of the disease. In the 1990s, researchers discovered two genes, known as BRCA1 and BRCA2, that are related to this family risk. A woman carrying mutations in these genes can have a risk as high as 90 percent of getting cancer. Women who test positive can opt for more frequent monitoring via mammogram screening, chemopreventive treatment with the drug tamoxifen, or even prophylactic removal of the breasts.

The HGP is accelerating knowledge on many disease genes— those involved in other cancers, heart disease, dementia, obesity, mental illness, and high blood pressure, for example. Increasingly, researchers are using DNA "chips" to carry out scans of the whole genome, which uncover many more genes linked with disease than known previously. However, many of these genes are far less predictive than BRCA1 and will contribute only a small amount to an individual's risk of disease. The challenge is to know how gene variants interact with environmental factors, like diet, and what can be done to mitigate overall risk.

Today genetics is leading the way to personalized medicine. Pharmacogenetics is the branch of genetics that looks at how an individual processes the drugs he or she is prescribed—whether his or her liver enzymes break them down too quickly, or not fast enough. Looking at a patient's genetic profile will enable doctors to determine which are the best drugs to prescribe and which are likely to cause side effects. Further advances are likely through the establishment of "biobanks," such as the UK Biobank, which is collecting DNA samples from populations in order to discover the distribution of genes that influence common diseases, so that new methods of diagnosis and treatment can be developed.

The Body

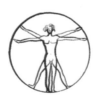

Oswald Avery

Oswald Avery was among the first molecular biologists to suggest that DNA played a significant role in the "transforming principle," which allowed dead bacteria to pass its virulent properties on to live bacteria. His research stimulated much interest in DNA and eventually led to the discovery that DNA carries the "life blueprint" for all living organisms.

Born: 1877, Halifax, Canada
Importance: one of the first molecular biologists to discover the properties of DNA
Died: 1955, Nashville, Tennessee

Born in Canada, Avery emigrated to New York at a young age and studied at Colgate University and then Columbia University, where he received a degree in medicine in 1904. Although he practiced medicine for a while, his real interest was research in microbiology. In 1913 he took up a position at the Rockefeller Institute, where he remained for the rest of his long career.

Avery's research interests focused on the microbes responsible for tuberculosis and pneumonia. He was intrigued by findings reported in 1928 by Fred Griffith, a public health microbiologist working in London. Griffith was working with pneumococci, one of the organisms that could cause pneumonia. There were two types of pneumococci, which Griffith called "rough" and "smooth" after the appearance of their colonies when grown on agar medium. The rough bacteria were innocuous, while the smooth ones were virulent. Their smooth appearance came from the presence of a carbohydrate "coat" around each microbe, which allowed them to evade the immune system and therefore cause disease.

When Griffith mixed live rough pneumococci with dead smooth pneumococci and injected the combination into lab mice, he found it was lethal. He said something, which he called the "transforming principle," had passed from the dead bacteria,

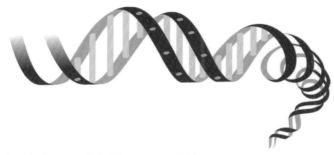

conferring its virulent properties upon the live bacteria. Avery set out to identify this transorming principle.

By the 1940s, it was known that chromosomes—tiny thread-like structures visible in the nucleus under a microscope—carried genetic information, a "blueprint" of the biochemical and physical characteristics of an organism, although it was not discovered how this worked until the 1960s. Chromosomes were composed of roughly half protein and half deoxyribonucleic acid (DNA). At the time, protein was considered the more significant part by biochemists, as it is more complex than DNA.

Avery spent years trying to pull the transforming principle out of his experimental mixtures in order to determine its chemical identity. He used enzymes to chop up various cell components: if an enzyme removed a cell component and the transforming property was retained in the experiment, then that component could be eliminated. In 1944 he and his colleagues, Colin McLeod and Maclyn Macarty, announced that DNA was the famous transforming principle. Scientists later found that DNA is the basis of all genes, carrying the life blueprint in all organisms from bacteria to humans. In 1953 Francis Crick and James Watson discovered the double-helix structure of DNA, which laid the foundations for an entirely new approach to medicine and biology.

The Body

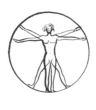

Francis Collins

Francis Collins investigated techniques for identifying potential disease genes within stretches of deoxyribonucleic acid (DNA). His approach, which came to be known as "positional cloning," has become the cornerstone of molecular genetics. Collins went on to lead the Human Genome Project (HGP), a multidisciplinary, international effort to map and sequence the human genetic blueprint.

Born: 1950, Staunton, Virgina
Importance: discovered many disease genes and oversaw the completion of the Human Genome Project

Collins initially preferred chemistry, regarding biology as "messy." He earned a degree in chemistry at the University of Virginia, then a PhD in physical chemistry at Yale. It was here that his interest in biochemistry was piqued. He developed a fascination for the molecules that carried the blueprint of life—DNA and the related ribonucleic acid (RNA). He decided to be part of the coming revolution in molecular biology and genetics and enrolled as a medical student at the University of North Carolina, earning his medical degree in 1977.

Between 1978 and 1981, Collins worked as a resident in internal medicine at the North Carolina Memorial Hospital. Returning to Yale, he took up a research position in genetics. It was here that he began to identify potential disease genes in DNA. The beauty of this positional cloning, for the researcher, lies in the way it allows the identification of a disease gene without necessarily having to know how it works (that can come later).

Collins's first success in this field was the identification of the gene for the lung disease cystic fibrosis in 1989. Later, he and his team uncovered the genes for Huntington's disease, neurofibromatosis, multiple endocrine neoplasia type 1, and a form of adult acute leukemia.

a political and religious conservative, and a Royalist. Over the next few years, he was active in research at the Société l'Ecole de Médecine and earned a post as a physician at the Salpêtrière Hospital. Following the restoration of the French throne, to Louis XVIII in 1815, Laënnec gained a position as Chief Physician to the Necker Hospital, through royal intervention.

At the time, auscultation involved the doctor laying his head on a patient's chest, while percussion involved tapping the chest, sometimes requiring the patient to bare the chest. In 1816, Laënnec had a young female patient who was too plump for auscultation and he had the idea of using a "mediator." He placed one end of a tightly rolled sheet of paper on her chest, and put his ear to the other. He found he heard the heartbeat much more clearly than he ever had by placing his ear directly against the chest.

Laënnec used his stethoscope to link chest sounds to a variety of heart and lung diseases, including asthma, pneumonia, and pleural effusion. In 1819, he published his book *On Mediate Auscultation*, which described 50 case histories in which chest sounds were linked to postmortem findings. Some physicians in Paris used the stethoscope to develop a new medical philosophy called "organicism," by which all disease could be identified through changes in the body's organs. For Laënnec's part, he believed the body to be composed of solid organs, fluids, and a life force. Disease, he said, was produced by a perturbation in any of the three. He argued that the life force was real, even though it could not be detected or measured. This was a controversial view. He also believed in the importance of emotional health and said, for instance, that tuberculosis resulted from poverty and its problems. Laënnec was influential, but never popular, among his peers. Following the second edition of his book on auscultation he moved back to his native Brittany, dying shortly thereafter of tuberculosis.

Epidemics and Pandemics

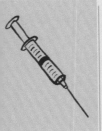

One of the earliest accounts of an epidemic appears in the writings of the Greek historian Thucydides and describes a mystery illness that swept Athens from 430 BC. The disease, which originated in Africa and spread through Persia to Greece, killed a quarter of the Athenian army, destroying the city's military ambitions, as well as exacting a huge toll of life among the civilian population. Today, the economy and infrastructure of many African countries have been wrecked by the HIV/AIDS pandemic. Meanwhile, many countries are stockpiling flu drugs and vaccines against a pandemic of avian influenza.

An epidemic is the occurrence of an unusually high number of cases of an infectious disease in an area (the term *outbreak* is often used for very localized epidemics). A pandemic is an epidemic with a global sweep, with the disease present in many, or even most, countries. The course of human history has been marked and changed by many epidemics. One of the most notable was the Black Death (1347–1351) when plague, carried by black rats, killed one third to one half of the entire population of Europe. This was the first of a wave of plague epidemics that continued to affect Europe well into the 17th century.

Armies and other population movements play an important role in spreading epidemics, particularly among nations with no immunity. The 15th century saw the European conquerors of the Americas introduce epidemic smallpox and other Western diseases to the native population. Killing millions, these epidemics must have played a role in weakening their resistance to invasion.

The flu pandemic of 1918–1919 killed between 20 and 40 million people—more people than were killed in the fighting of World War I. One fifth of the world's population was affected, and the life expectancy of Americans lowered for a decade afterwards. Smaller flu pandemics occurred in 1957 and 1968.

Influenza is a bird disease with the responsible viruses mutated so that humans become susceptible. Flu outbreaks occur annually, with the virus responsible being slightly different in its genetic makeup each time. The H5N1 strain of bird flu was discovered in 2003 and 2004 in Southeast Asia. In some affected flocks, all the birds have died. The disease is transmissible to humans, particularly in places where there is close contact between people and chickens. Out of the 385 reported cases, 243 people have died from H5N1 flu, which makes this an unusually lethal form of the disease. Two of the conditions for a pandemic are already fulfilled by H5N1 bird flu: It is a previously unknown strain of the disease, so there is no natural immunity; and it is a zoonosis (a disease transmissible from other species—in this case birds—to humans). The third criterion for a pandemic, that the disease is also readily transmissible between humans, has not yet been fulfilled. However, flu mutates remarkably rapidly and it may be just a matter of time before H5N1 acquires the mutation that will make it infectious enough to trigger a pandemic.

For this reason, the World Health Organization (WHO) is coordinating intensive surveillance so that outbreaks of infection are dealt with and contained before they can escalate to pandemic, or even epidemic, level. Governments are building up supplies of antiflu drugs and prepandemic vaccines, although there will be a delay of four to six months between a pandemic strain's appearance and the manufacture of a vaccine able to tackle it.

Just as the armies of the past spread disease by marching into new countries, so our modern lifestyles threaten to increase the incidence of pandemic disease. Increased international travel, more contact between humans and animals, and global warming are significant factors contributing to the risk of pandemics.

John Snow

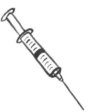

Taking a scientific approach to medicine, John Snow's ideas were ahead of his time. His work on the causes and spread of cholera, in particular, was groundbreaking, and it was almost certainly his insight that brought an end to major outbreaks of the disease in Britain. Furthermore, his ideas on prevention of infection are still effective today, proving that, even with vaccination and antibiotics, regular hand-washing and the avoidance of contaminated food and water are vital in stopping the spread of disease.

Born: 1813, York, England
Importance: his work on cholera was an important milestone in the development of epidemiology, the science of the causes and spread of disease; pioneered use of anesthesia in England
Died: 1858, London, England

Snow became apprenticed to a surgeon in Newcastle upon Tyne at the age of 14. In 1831, while still an apprentice, he was sent to help deal with the first outbreak of cholera in England, in the port of Sutherland. He studied medicine in London from 1836, and gained a post at the Westminster Hospital. He was elected to the Royal College of Surgeons in 1838 and to the Royal College of Physicians in 1850.

Snow believed in the germ theory, rather than the idea that disease was spread through "miasma" or bad air. He also proposed that cholera was transmitted through contaminated water and that its cause was some kind of organism. Snow investigated the transmission of cholera during the 1848 epidemic in London, publishing his findings in his classic work *On the Mode of Communication of Cholera*, on August 29, 1849. He then worked on an outbreak occurring in August 1854, in the area in and around Broad Street, near his own home in central London.

He produced a map, now famous, that traced this cholera outbreak to the water supplied by the Broad Street pump, where the well was located close to a sewage pipe. He found in the case

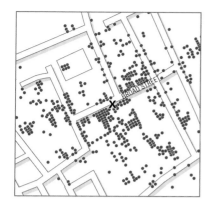

X Pump
• Deaths from cholera

Left: In 1848, Snow mapped a cholera outbreak near his home in London, showing the deaths were concentrated around the water pump on Broad Street. This indicated the source of the outbreak was contaminated water from that particular pump.

of deaths located closer to another street pump, the families either preferred to get their water from the Broad Street pump, or the victims were children who went to school near the Broad Street pump. He recommended the removal of the pump handle, so the well could no longer be used, an intervention often said to have stopped the Broad Street outbreak although, in fact, it was already waning according to data collected at the time. His theory on the transmission of cholera—from person to person—became accepted, however, and his work saved the lives of thousands. He became an influential figure, being elected as President of the Medical Society of London in 1855.

Snow was also interested in the science of breathing. Ether was introduced into England as an anesthetic in 1846 and chloroform in 1847. Snow devised inhalation devices for them and also developed a theory that listed five stages of anesthesia. He became England's first expert anesthetist and administered chloroform to Queen Victoria during the birth of Prince Leopold, her eighth child, in 1853. This led to the acceptance of anesthesia in medicine. Victoria also used anesthesia for the birth of her next, and final, child—Princess Beatrice—in 1857. The next year Snow suffered a stroke while working in his office and died shortly afterward.

Disease

Louis Pasteur

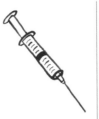

Considered the father of microbiology, Louis Pasteur is perhaps best known for the pasteurization process to which he gave his name and for his pioneering work in the field of vaccination. He also developed the practice of sterilizing medical equipment in boiling water, which he called for in 1874.

Born: 1822, Dôle, France
Importance: founded the science of microbiology and the germ theory of disease; made important discoveries in chemistry and immunology
Died: 1895, Paris, France

Pasteur attended the Ecole Normale Supérieure, the main science school in Paris, where he developed an interest in chemistry. In 1848, he became a Professor of Chemistry at the University of Strasbourg, later moving to take up a position at the University of Lille. He made the transition from chemistry to biology (although he always took a chemical approach to scientific problems) through work on fermentation in connection with the wine and beer industry, showing that fermentation was caused by microbes.

Pasteur returned to Paris in 1857, becoming director of scientific studies at the Ecole Normale Supérieure. Ten years later, he became Professor of Chemistry at the Sorbonne. In the 1860s, he carried out classic experiments showing that life did not arise from spontaneous generation, as some had previously believed. These involved placing a sterile fermentation broth in a special flask with an "S"-shaped or "swan" neck. Because of its design, contamination could not enter the broth and it remained sterile. As soon as the neck was broken, the broth started to putrefy, as microbes from the air entered and began to multiply.

This led Pasteur to develop the pasteurization process, in which brief, moderate heating destroys the microbes in milk, wine, and other substances, stopping them from spoiling. This helped stop the spread of tuberculosis and typhoid through contaminated milk. He continued his work in microbiology, investigating the causes of diseases in animals, then humans. One of his first studies involved a bacterial disease of silkworms, which was devastating the silk industry in France. He also studied microbial diseases in pigs, cattle, and poultry and identified important *Streptococcus* and *Staphylococcus* species that cause human disease.

The concept of vaccination had already been developed by Edward Jenner with his work on smallpox (see page 46). In the late 1870s, Pasteur developed the idea using the chicken cholera bacillus. He found that if the bacillus was aged, it lost much of its infective power, but was able to confer some protection against the disease when injected. In 1881, he performed a dramatic public experiment with a crude anthrax vaccine, injecting it into a group of 25 sheep, cows, and goats, while a control group did not receive the vaccine. Then, all animals were infected with anthrax. None of the vaccinated group succumbed to the disease. He then began work on a rabies vaccine, based upon the dried spinal cord of a rabid rabbit. He was able to show that it could save guinea pigs and rabbits that had been exposed to infected saliva.

> "Where observation is concerned, chance favors only the prepared mind."
>
> Louis Pasteur

Understandably, Pasteur was wary of extending this work to humans. In 1885, however, he treated a nine-year-old boy, Joseph Meister, who had been bitten by a rabid dog. The boy survived (and went on to become a caretaker at the Pasteur Institute). The following year, Pasteur vaccinated more than 2,500 people who had been infected with rabies and only a handful of them died of the disease. Such was Pasteur's fame that a public subscription was set up to open the first Pasteur Institute in Paris in 1888.

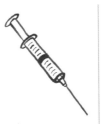

Champion of Bacteriology

Robert Koch

Building on foundations set by Louis Pasteur (see page 54), Robert Koch firmly established germ theory as a credible science. He made a number of significant discoveries in the causes of infectious diseases, identifying the causative agents of anthrax, tuberculosis, and cholera, among others. Famously, in 1882, Koch proposed a number of postulates relating to infectious diseases, which are still used today when investigating their causes.

Born: 1843, Clausthal, Germany
Importance: pioneer of modern medical microbiology; founded principles of infectious disease
Died: 1910, Baden-Baden, Germany

Robert Koch trained in medicine in Göttingen, Germany, graduating in 1866. His interest in bacteriology began with his work on anthrax, a highly contagious cattle disease, which can also spread to humans. In 1877, he discovered that the disease was caused by the microbe *Bacillus anthracis*. In doing so, he made the important discovery that anthrax bacilli can form spores—a dormant form resistant to heat and drying—which can survive for many years in soil and can also become airborne and travel great distances. Koch claimed this was the underlying cause of many apparently inexplicable outbreaks of the disease, for under certain conditions, the bacilli may reactivate from the spore form. Koch isolated anthrax bacilli from infected cows and produced a laboratory culture of these bacteria capable of causing the disease. This was a key experiment in the development of medical microbiology.

In 1882 he identified the tubercle bacillus, *Mycobacterium tuberculosis*, responsible for tuberculosis (TB). He gained international renown for his work and began traveling widely to study infection. In 1883, in Egypt, he identified *Cholera vibrio*, the bacterium that causes cholera (unknown to Koch, the

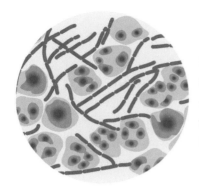

Left: Koch's examination of anthrax bacilli, which appear under the microscope as tiny, rod-like structures, was one of the pioneering developments in the field of microbiology.

organism had previously been discovered in 1854 by the Italian Filippo Pacini, whose work was ignored as the germ theory had not yet become established).

Koch made significant technical advances in microbiology. He used dyes to stain bacterial preparations for easier microscope study, and used agar gel, a solid medium, to culture bacteria, gaining better results than with the liquid medium previously favored. His assistant, Julius Richard Petri, designed a glass dish used to incubate and grow bacterial colonies for study. The Petri dish, now usually made of plastic, is still widely used by biologists. Koch also showed steam was more effective than boiling water for sterilizing surgical equipment.

Koch's *The Aetiology of Traumatic Infectious Diseases* was published in 1879, and in 1884 he formulated his postulates: first, the causative microbe must be present in all cases of the disease; second, it must be possible to create a pure culture of this organism; third, this culture, grown through many generations of the microbe, must be capable of reproducing the disease if injected into an experimental animal; and fourth, the organism must be capable of being isolated again from the inoculated animal.

Koch tried to build on his TB research by developing a vaccine called tuberculin. This was not very successful, although it survives as a method of determining whether someone has actually been exposed to TB. In 1905, Koch was awarded the Nobel Prize for his work on TB.

Disease

Marie Curie

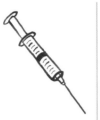

Marie Curie was the first woman to receive a Nobel Prize and the only to hold Nobel Prizes for two sciences. Through her pioneering work in radioactivity, she discovered new elements polonium and radium, paving the way for radiation biology and radiotherapy treatment in cancer.

Born: Marie Sklodowska, 1867, Warsaw, Poland
Importance: discovered polonium and radium, thereby pioneering the use of radiation in medicine
Died: 1934, Sallanches, France

Marie Sklodowska grew up in Russian-dominated Poland and, after working as a governess to earn money to support her own and her sister, Bronya's, studies, went to the Sorbonne in Paris to study physics. She graduated first in her class in 1891 and went on to study mathematics. In 1895 she married Pierre Curie, whom she met at the Sorbonne.

In 1896, French physicist Henri Becquerel (1852–1908) discovered radioactivity and Curie decided to work on this for her doctoral degree. She discovered that radioactivity was an atomic property of the element uranium and that the element thorium also emitted radioactivity. The mineral pitchblende was more radioactive than its known uranium and thorium content suggested and she set out to discover its other radioactive elements. Pierre gave up his own research and in July 1898 they isolated polonium, a new element that Marie named after her native country. In December they also isolated radium. Working in an old shed under very difficult conditions, the couple went on to purify one tenth of a gram of radium chloride from a ton of pitchblende. The radium had extraordinary properties—it evolved heat and glowed in the dark.

In 1903, Marie Curie received the first PhD ever to be awarded to a woman in France. In the same year, she and Pierre shared the Nobel Prize for Physics with Henri Becquerel for their research on radioactivity. The potential of radium as a cancer treatment was soon realized. Radium tubes, capsules, and needles were easier to use in therapy than X-ray machines, and the Radium Institute of Paris was opened just before World War I. Fund-raising efforts were launched, for radium was one of the most expensive substances in the world.

In 1906, Pierre Curie died in a road accident. Marie took over his post at the Sorbonne and, by 1910, she was Professor of Physics and head of the faculty of physics at the Sorbonne, the first woman ever to hold such a high academic post in France. She devoted much of her time to supervising students and raising research funds. In 1911, she was awarded the Nobel Prize for Chemistry.

> "It is easy to understand how important for me is the conviction that our discovery is a blessing for humankind, not only by its scientific importance, but also because it permits to reduce human suffering and treat a terrible disease. This is, indeed, a great reward for the years of our enormous effort."
>
> Marie Curie

During World War I, Curie organized mobile X-ray services for military hospitals, even driving one of the mobile X-ray vans, known as "little Curies." After the war, she visited the United States many times and in 1921, the women of America collected enough money for Curie to purchase a gram of radium for her research. Meanwhile, fund-raising efforts in Poland helped her realize her dream of opening a Radium Institute in Warsaw.

Marie Curie was one of many who suffered health problems from working with radioactive elements, and she died of aplastic anemia at the age of 67.

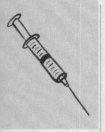

Germ Theory of Disease

Infectious diseases such as typhoid, cholera, plague, and smallpox claimed millions of lives before doctors realized that the causative agents were microbes (viruses, bacteria, fungi, or protozoa). The term "germ" is often used to describe a harmful microbe, for many microbes are harmless or even beneficial. The "germ theory" of disease, put forward by Robert Koch in the mid-19th century, is one of the great milestones in medical history.

Previously fever, one of the main symptoms of infection, had been thought to arise from various causes, chief of which was exposure to "miasma" or bad air. Similarly, doctors had no scientific explanation for diseases like typhoid; there was no awareness of the role of contaminated food and water.

The French chemist, Louis Pasteur, carried out groundbreaking work that was, eventually, to change the miasma theory (see page 54). He studied putrefaction in brewing and winemaking and then devised an elegant series of experiments to show that microbes in the air were the cause of changes that occured. From there, it was just a short step to the conclusion that microbes might play a role in certain diseases and their transmission. Pasteur turned his attention to a disease among silkworms that was devastating the French silk industry and showed that bacteria were responsible for the disease. He then looked at the role of microbes in a range of animal diseases. He was particularly interested in anthrax and rabies and extended his ideas about microbial causes to develop vaccines for these diseases in the late 19th century.

However, it was Koch who actually formulated the germ theory, putting forward his ideas in his classic work *The Aetiology of Traumatic Infectious Diseases* in 1879 (see page 56).

Koch's postulates, derived from experiments he had carried out on isolating and growing up pure cultures of various bacteria, are still used in microbiology laboratories today to investigate the causes of outbreaks of disease and epidemics.

Koch discovered the tuberculosis bacillus in 1882 and the cholera bacillus in 1883. His contemporaries went on to isolate the microbes that caused many common diseases such as typhoid, pneumonia, leprosy, whooping cough, plague, and syphilis.

Bacillus: A rod-shaped bacterium, such as *Bacillus anthracis*, the cause of anthrax, belonging to the Bacillus genus (the classification above species, below family).

Germ theory also drove the development of vaccines and, later, antibiotics such as penicillin and streptomycin. Vaccination eradicated smallpox from the world in the late 1970s and has almost achieved the eradication of polio. Meanwhile, new threats have emerged with HIV/AIDS, severe acute respiratory syndrome (SARS), and H5NI avian influenza. Identifying the causative organism through careful laboratory work has formed the basis for developing drugs and vaccines against these infectious diseases.

The germ theory has also proved useful in understanding diseases not usually perceived as infections. For instance, viruses can sometimes play a role in cancer. Cervical cancer has been shown to have a very strong association with infection with the human papilloma virus (HPV). A vaccine against HPV has been found to provide a very high degree of protection against this form of cancer and the vaccine is now being made generally available to girls and young women. And the bacterium *Helicobacter pylori* has been shown to play a role in the development of peptic ulcers and stomach cancer. Its eradication with antibiotics is now seen as an important component of treatment for these conditions.

Disease

Frederick Banting

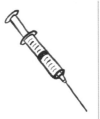

In 1923, Frederick Banting was awarded a Nobel Prize for his groundbreaking work in the field of diabetes. Together with student Charles Best, Banting found a way of extracting insulin in order to treat the disease—at the time, fatal without treatment or cure. Today, millions of people owe their lives to his pioneering work.

Born: 1891, Alliston, Ontario
Importance: extracted insulin, providing the first treatment for people with diabetes
Died: 1941, Newfoundland, Canada

Diabetes is one of the most common chronic diseases, and carries a high risk of complications such as blindness, heart disease, and poor circulation in the legs, which may lead to amputation. There are two forms of the disease. In type 1 diabetes, which people are usually born with, the pancreas does not produce the hormone insulin. In type 2 diabetes, the body is resistant to insulin, so cannot make use of it. Type 2 diabetes is on the increase, as the population ages and more people become obese, which is a risk factor for the disease. The pancreas produces insulin after a meal and helps to store excess glucose from food in the liver. Without insulin, blood glucose levels remain high which is damaging to the heart and other parts of the body in the long term.

Frederick Banting worked as an orthopedic surgeon in London, Ontario. He had long been interested in the plight of people with diabetes. Much was already known of the underlying cause—a lack of insulin. The hormone had even been named and it was known that it was produced in the pancreas by clusters of cells called the islets of Langherans. What was difficult was extracting the insulin in a form that could be given to patients, as enzymes in the pancreas tended to destroy it before it could be isolated and purified.

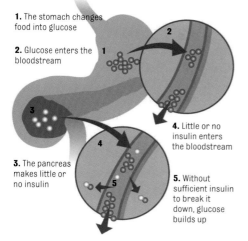

1. The stomach changes food into glucose

2. Glucose enters the bloodstream

3. The pancreas makes little or no insulin

4. Little or no insulin enters the bloodstream

5. Without sufficient insulin to break it down, glucose builds up

Left: In Type 1 diabetes, the pancreas makes little or no insulin, and so cannot break down the glucose in the bloodstream. Morton's discovery allowed patients to be injected with insulin directly.

In 1920, Banting came up with the idea of tying off the pancreatic ducts, surgically, to deactivate the enzymes and thereby preserve the insulin content. He and Best, he began experimenting on ten dogs in May 1921 and by August had obtained some insulin from the islets of Langherans (the name insulin comes from the latin word for "island"). They administered their insulin to the dogs, which had abnormally high glucose levels, and found the levels normalized. Later, with the help of chemist James Betram Collip, they were able to purify the insulin and soon had enough to commence human clinical trials.

The medical world was quick to recognize the significance of this work, awarding both Banting and Best with the Nobel Prize for Physiology or Medicine. For many years, insulin was extracted from pig pancreas but now human insulin for treatment can be produced through genetic engineering.

Insulin is a treatment for diabetes, not a cure. There has also been some success in transplantation of islet cells. The next step forward could be to transplant insulin-producing pancreatic cells derived from human stem cells, which might provide a permanent cure for those with type 1 diabetes.

Disease

Alfred Blalock and Helen Taussig

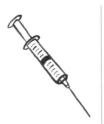

In 1945, Alfred Blalock and Helen Taussig of Johns Hopkins University carried out the first operation to correct a congenital heart defect, thereby offering new hope to "blue babies" and their families. The advance marked the beginning of the modern era of cardiac surgery, which, today, can cure or alleviate many different heart conditions that were previously fatal.

Born: (Blalock) 1899, Culloden, Georgia; (Taussig) 1898, Cambridge, Massachusetts

Importance: pioneered operation to save lives of "blue babies"

Died: (Blalock) 1964, Baltimore, Ohio; (Taussig) 1986, Kennett Square, Pennsylvania

Prior to the 1940s, babies born with congenital heart defects did not usually survive. When the heart does not work properly, the blood cannot be oxygenated. Therefore, such children tend to have a bluish tinge to their skin known as cyanosis (oxygenated blood is pink) and are known as "blue babies."

A heart surgeon, Alfred Blalock began his career with research into shock brought on by blood loss and trauma. He showed that blood transfusion was an effective treatment in such cases, an approach that saved thousands of lives during World War II. Ably assisted by technician Vivien Thomas, whose contribution is often overlooked, Blalock carried out work on dogs, developing new surgical techniques that he would later use to perform the blue-baby operations. In one animal in particular, they carried out an anastomosis—surgical joining—between the left subclavian artery (which supplies blood to the neck and arms) and the left pulmonary artery. This procedure was to prove crucial in the success of the blue-baby operation.

Blalock teamed up with Helen Taussig, who had a long-standing interest in a congenital heart condition called tetralogy

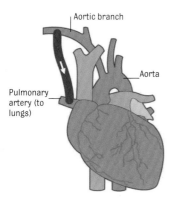

Left: In a Blalock-Taussig shunt, now modified from the original method, an artificial tube (shown in dark red) diverts blood from the aorta directly into the pulmonary artery, thus bypassing the defects caused by blue-baby syndrome and allowing blood to receive oxygen from the lungs.

of Fallot. As the name suggests, this particular blue-baby syndrome involves four defects: there is narrowing of the artery serving the lungs; a hole in the wall between the two lower chambers of the heart (ventricles); enlargement of the right ventricle; and defective positioning of the aorta, which is the main artery to the body.

Blalock and Taussig believed that the former's new surgical techniques could bypass the defects, allowing the affected baby's blood a new passage to oxygenation. Their first patient, in 1945, was 15-month-old Eileen Saxon. The operation was a success, with baby Eileen becoming less and less blue in the days that followed. By 1952, the team had performed over 1,000 such operations and surgeons from all over the world traveled to Johns Hopkins to learn the techniques.

Both physicians were honored nationally and internationally for their contribution to cardiology—a superb example of how experimental work can be translated into benefit for the patient.

Disease

Archie Cochrane

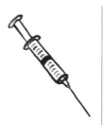

Archibald Cochrane was a staunch pioneer of the randomized clinical trial, in which active treatment is compared with a placebo (dummy) treatment. Now regarded as the "gold standard" in medical research, Cochrane carried out many such trials on pharmaceutical, surgical, and other healthcare interventions. He also set up an epidemiology unit for the Medical Research Council (MRC), establishing a worldwide reputation for its work on the causes and natural history of anemia, asthma, glaucoma, and other diseases.

Born: 1909, Galashiels, Scotland

Importance: pioneered the use of randomized controlled clinical trials

Died: 1988, Holt, England

Cochrane graduated in science from Cambridge in 1922. He also studied medicine and did research in tissue culture at the Strangeways Laboratory in Cambridge. However, he became disenchanted with this work and developed psychological problems, seeking treatment through psychoanalysis in Berlin, Vienna, and The Hague. Returning to Britain in 1934, he became a medical student at University College, London. He interrupted his studies to serve as a volunteer in the Spanish Civil War but resumed in 1937, receiving his degree in 1938.

After the war, Cochrane trained in preventive medicine. One of his major influences was the teaching of Bradford Hill in epidemiology and randomized clinical trials. He continued his training in Philadelphia and became interested in X-ray studies of tuberculosis. These films were examined by different people or by the same people at different times and Cochrane developed ideas about inter-observer and intra-observer error, which could influence the interpretation of data.

In 1948, Cochrane joined the Medical Research Council

(MRC) Pneumoconiosis Research Unit in Cardiff. He was to work on this lung disease for over a decade, developing a system of classifying X-rays of coal workers according to their exposure to coal dust and their level of disability. He continued this involvement with follow-up studies of the population of Rhondda Fach (the "two valleys" which gave the study its name). Cochrane moved epidemiology forward —he believed in getting the highest possible response rate in surveys and follow-up studies. In recognition of his achievements, the MRC asked him to set up a new epidemiology unit in Cardiff in 1960. In the same year, he became Professor in Tuberculosis and Diseases of the Chest at the Welsh National School of Medicine.

> "It is surely a great criticism of our profession that we have not organized a critical summary, by speciality or subspeciality, adapated periodically, of all relevant randomized controlled trials."
>
> Archie Cochrane

Cochrane wrote the influential book *Effectiveness and Efficiency: Random Reflections on Health Services*, published in 1972. This volume stressed the importance of using medical interventions so that they are more likely to do good than harm. It also forms the basis of what we now call evidence-based medicine, where doctors are encouraged to take a more rational, and cost-effective, approach to their prescribing. In response to Cochrane's views on randomized controlled trials, the Cochrane Collaboration was formed a few years after his death. Around 10,000 medical experts worldwide conduct detailed reviews of medical treatments so patients can be offered those that have the best evidence base. The reviews are published electronically in *The Cochrane Database of Systematic Reviews*.

Austin Bradford Hill

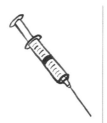

An expert on the application of statistics in epidemiology, Austin Bradford Hill, along with colleague Richard Doll, carried out a large prospective study on smoking and lung cancer. Taking over 34,000 British doctors born between 1900 and 1930, they established a definite link between smoking and lung cancer. This had a powerful effect on public health policy, starting a trend that has recently seen smoking banned in public places in many countries.

Born: 1897, London, England
Importance: pioneer in applying statistics to medicine and, with Richard Doll, demonstrated the dangers to health of smoking
Died: 1991, Windemere, England

Hill was the third son of Sir Leonard Erskine Hill, FRS, Professor of Physiology at the London Hospital, and had an early ambition to study medicine. He served as a pilot in World War I but contracted tuberculosis and was invalided out. The time lost in hospital and convalescence made it impractical for him to study medicine so he graduated in economics instead. He joined the statistics group at the National Institute of Medical Research in north London, in 1923. He then moved to the London School of Hygiene and Tropical Medicine, joining the medical statistician Major Greenwood, a friend of his father's, who had also been one of his teachers. His career progressed and he became Professor of Medical Statistics there in 1947, succeeding Major Greenwood.

In 1948, the Medical

"To anyone involved in medical statistics, epidemiology, or public health, Bradford Hill was simply the world's leading medical statistician."

Peter Armitage, Hill's successor at the London School of Hygiene and Tropical Medicine

Research Council (MRC) was offered a small amount of the antibiotic streptomycin to treat patients with tuberculosis (TB). There was not enough of the new drug to distribute generally, so the MRC recruited Hill to advise them. He declared the only ethical way forward was to set up a clinical trial in which one group received streptomycin and the other received standard treatment. This was the first randomized controlled trial in human subjects (although the method was used in agricultural research) and it was to become a model for clinical research from then on.

Epidemiology: The study of patterns of disease in a population and the various risk factors involved.

In 1948 Hill and Richard Doll (then a young doctor working for the MRC and later professor of medicine at Oxford) carried out a survey of patients in 20 London hospitals. Their case-control study, published in 1950, established cigarette smoking as a cause of lung cancer. The medical establishment received the results with some skepticism, however, so Hill and Doll decided to carry out their much larger study, involving the 34,000 doctors, in order to confirm their conclusions.

Between 1950 and 1952, Hill was president of the Royal Statistical Society. He became a Fellow of the Royal Society in 1954 and, on his retirement in 1961, he was knighted. He published an important textbook, *Principles of Medical Statistics*, in 1937, which went through 11 editions during his lifetime. Doll continued the work on the doctors' study and, 50 years after it began, was able to show that doctors born between 1900 and 1930 who continued to smoke would lose, on average, 10 years of life to smoking-related disease. Those doctors who gave up were shown to gain back some, or all, of these lost years, depending on the age at which they quit.

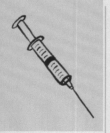

Stem Cells and Cloning

In 1968, the first stem-cell transplant was performed at the University of Minnesota when a four-month-old boy received an infusion of bone marrow. The child had severe combined immune deficiency (SCID), a rare inherited disorder, which left him completely vulnerable to infection as his immune system lacked lymphocytes and could not, therefore, make antibodies against invading organisms.

Bone marrow contains cells that can turn into lymphocytes to replace the deficiency in this disease. The first operation was successful and has been followed by thousands of bone-marrow transplants for SCID and related diseases. The hope now is that stem cells can be used as a treatment for many other conditions, such as diabetes, stroke, heart attack, and Parkinson's disease.

Stem cells have two important properties that distinguish them from other kinds of cells: they can proliferate, possibly indefinitely, while still staying as stem cells, and they can also spontaneously change—a process known as differentiation—into one or more new cell types under the right conditions. Therefore they have the potential to provide an unlimited supply of cells for repairing different parts of the body.

It has long been clear that there must be stem cells in the body, because three billion cells (out of an approximate total of 50 million million) die each minute and are presumably replaced from some kind of reserve. In 1998, James Thomson of the University of Wisconsin announced the establishment of a stable line of human embryonic stem cells (hESCs), derived from cells taken from the inner cell mass (100 to 150 cells) of a week-old human embryo. These were grown in culture with an appropriate mix of nutrients and growth culture. Once established, a "line" of hESCs is essentially immortal and may be frozen for storage in a cell bank. Researchers make a distinction between ESCs and stem cells from other sources—often referring to the latter as somatic stem cells—claiming that ESCs have the ability to differentiate into many more cell types than do somatic stem cells.

The developing fetus—between four and 12 weeks—is a rich source of stem cells. Exploiting their use has not yet occurred, because of the difficulties of obtaining the cells and ethical considerations around using aborted fetuses for medical purposes. Many types of tissue-specific stem cells, such as nerve stem cells, have been found in fetal tissue. Cord stem cells, which are a type of blood stem cell, are found in the umbilical cord and placenta of a newborn baby. Finally, some parts of the body, such as the skin, liver, and even the brain, have so-called tissue specific or adult stem cells, which help renew and replace old cells. Generally adult stem cells only differentiate into their tissue of origin, although research has shown that bone-marrow cells can form other cell types, such as cartilage and maybe even heart muscle cells.

Cloning, the process used to create Dolly the sheep, could be another source of stem cells. If a somatic cell—a skin cell for instance—is transferred into an empty egg and treated so as to reprogram its genes, the result would be an embryo that is a clone, or copy, of the original cell and a source of stem cells for the person who donated it. This would sidestep any problem relating to rejection of stem cells for treatment that had been donated from someone else. This approach is called "therapeutic cloning" and it is different from "reproductive cloning," in which a whole cloned organism is grown from the embryo. Human reproductive cloning is banned in most countries and therapeutic cloning is probably a long way off, owing to a shortage of human eggs for research like this and the ethical concerns about using animal eggs for this purpose.

Luc Montagnier

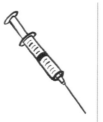

In 1982, already well known for his work on viruses and how they interact with their host organism, researcher Luc Montagnier was called upon by doctors at the Hôpital Bichat, in Paris, to investigate the AIDS epidemic. By May 1983, he reported the discovery of a virus that he believed was the cause of AIDS, and subsequently went on to make other discoveries that were to prove invaluable in understanding how HIV infects people, saving the lives of many in the process.

Born: 1932, Chabris, France
Importance: together with American virologist Robert Gallo, discovered the human immunodeficiency virus, opening up the way for treatment of HIV/AIDS

AIDS (acquired immunodeficiency syndrome) was first noticed by the medical community when eight cases of Kaposi's sarcoma (KS), a rare skin cancer, were noted among young homosexual men in New York in just one year (1981). At the same time, there was a sudden increase in cases of an unusual lung infection called *Pneumocystis carinii pneumonia* (PCP) in both Los Angeles and New York.

At first it was believed only gay men were at risk, but soon cases of PCP were found among drug users and the disease also appeared in the UK. Both KS and PCP occur when the immune system protecting the body from infection is severely weakened, so it appeared the new disease undermined immunity. In August 1982, doctors began to call the disease AIDS and by 1983 disease was present in the US, Canada, fifteen European countries, Haiti, Zaire, seven Latin American countries, Australia, and Japan.

Montagnier studied science at the University of Poitiers and qualified in medicine from the University of Paris. In 1974, he became Research Director at the Centre National de la Recherche Scientifique and moved to the Pasteur Institute in 1985.

In May 1983, while working for the Hôpital Bichat, Montagnier reported the discovery of lymphadenopathy-associated virus (LAV), which he believed probably caused AIDS. His team sent a sample of the virus to the Centers for Disease Control (CDC) in the US for further study. A year later, Robert Gallo announced the discovery of a virus he called HTLV-III (human T-cell leukemia/lymphoma virus) which he also claimed to be the cause of AIDS. Gallo's team found HTLV-III in the CD4 cells of more than 50 patients who had AIDS and also in some healthy individuals who were at high risk of developing the disease. They also found antibodies against the virus in the blood of infected people and developed methods for growing the viruses in cells, so that further experiments could be done.

There was controversy over whether Gallo's HTLV-III had come from the LAV sample that Montagnier had sent to the US. It was not clear whether Gallo discovered HIV (human immunodeficiency virus, as it came to be known) independently, or whether he "rediscovered" the virus in Montagnier's sample.

Montagnier and Gallo eventually agreed that LAV and HTLV-III were the same virus and the two men are now usually given joint credit for its discovery. Later, researchers sequenced the genome of HIV, which meant it was possible to compare HIV with other viruses and learn more about how it infected cells. It also provided a starting point for making drugs that would stop the infection. Montagnier went on to found the World Foundation for AIDS Research and Prevention and has received many awards, including the French Légion d'Honneur.

Thanks to the basis provided by Montagnier and Gallo's work, HIV/AIDS can be treated by drugs that block the life cycle of the virus, usually administered in a combination called "highly active antretroviral therapy," meaning it is no longer a death sentence but a chronic disease.

Paracelsus

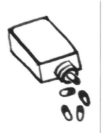

Were he alive today, Renaissance physician Paracelsus would be considered an eccentric practitioner of alternative medicine-cum-faith healer, and would be dismissed as a crank by the scientific orthodoxy. Yet "miraculous" cures were attributed to him. He has been described as "the most original medical theoretician of Renaissance Europe" and "the great medical pioneer of his age," and his name lives on.

Born: 1493, Einsiedeln, Switzerland

Importance: alchemist and physician whose holistic approach to health is reflected in alternative medicine today

Died: 1541, Salzburg, Austria

Paracelsus was the adopted name of Phillip von Hohenheim, a celebrated physician and occultist. He received his preliminary medical education from his father, also a physician, and studied at Ferrara, claiming that he obtained his doctor's degree there, although there is no evidence to support this.

In 1527, Paracelsus was summoned by the town council of Basel to help deal with a syphilis epidemic. He went on to become town physician and a university lecturer there. His behavior, however, outraged the authorities: he burned the books of Galen and Avicenna (the medical orthodoxy of the time, see pages 16 and 20) and wore laborer's clothes in the street instead of the robes of office. Hated by his colleagues, he was known as the "the wild ass of Einsiedeln." He soon left Basel, and spent the rest of his life traveling and practicing, undertaking hazardous journeys throughout Europe, Russia, and possibly Asia Minor and Africa, seeking hidden medical knowledge.

Paracelsus was a prolific writer. Around 1531, philosophical treatises began to appear in addition to the medical ones, and we can assume that this development arose from his experiences during his travels. Although his ideas are sometimes obscure, they can be generally described as Hermetic, pagan, and animistic, showing him as an alchemist, astrologer, faith healer, and pagan philosopher. At times he was accused, with some justification, of practising magic. Named by his peers the "Luther of medicine," he is perhaps remembered as much for his personality as his medical achievements. He had a quarrelsome temperament and a hatred of academic physicians and medical authorities.

Paracelsus was an expert in the application of herbal remedies and also pioneered the use of chemistry in medicine, using mineral acids, inorganic salts, and alchemical procedures in making remedies. He was the first known person to investigate the use of opium as a painkiller and introduced a version of laudanum (a tincture of opium) to the medical world. He made a significant contribution to the field of toxicology, recognizing that toxic substances could be helpful in small doses, a discovery that anticipated later developments in the field of immunization.

> "The physician should know what is above nature, what is above species, what is above life, what the visible is and the invisible."
>
> Paracelsus

A spiritual philosophy underpinned Paracelsus's work: he believed that a human being was a soul and a spirit as well as a body and, therefore, that an illness of the body might have a non-physical cause. He believed that there were realms of existence beyond the physical world (see quote above). Above all, Paracelsus believed that nature was the best healer and that the doctor's task was to cooperate with, and facilitate, natural processes. He also had an early insight into the psychological aspects of illness, referring in his writing to unconscious fantasies as an etiological factor. It could be therefore be argued that his treatments included a psychotherapeutic aspect, and thus that he anticipated modern psychoanalysis.

William Withering

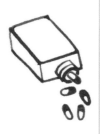

Through his study of digitalis, a drug extracted from the foxglove, Withering developed the first scientific framework for the discovery and development of drugs. Today, around half of all medicines are derived from plant sources, and the principles by which their dosing, efficacy, and toxicity are investigated are broadly similar to those that Withering employed.

Born: 1741, Wellington, England

Importance: laid the groundwork for modern pharmacology with his studies on digitalis, the active ingredient of the foxglove

Died: 1799, Sparkbrook, England

The son of an apothecary, Withering came from a medical family and studied medicine in Edinburgh, graduating in 1766. He went into practice in Stafford and then moved to Birmingham. He saw poor patients free of charge but also had a lucrative private practice. Withering was a man of wide interests. He shared an enthusiasm for botany with his wife, Helena. In 1776, he produced a book called *The Botanical Arrangement of All the Vegetables Naturally Growing in Great Britain*, which went into 14 editions over the subsequent 100 years. He was elected a Fellow of the Linnean Society in 1789.

Withering was active in the Lunar Society of Birmingham, where he met the great chemist, Joseph Priestley, and other influential men of science. Interested in chemistry, he carried out work analyzing the mineral content of different waters, as well as developing a standard test for the presence of sulphates. He was well known in Europe: a French botanist named a genus of plants after him (*Witheringia solanacea*) and a German geologist gave his name to the mineral witherite. He became a Fellow of the Royal Society in 1784, still the highest honor bestowed on a British scientist.

Withering's most significant legacy was in the field of drugs. On hearing about a herbal tea containing foxgloves that a Shropshire woman used for curing dropsy (a swelling of the ankles), he carried out a study of its various ingredients. Foxgloves (*Digitalis purpurea*) have a long history in medicine, but Withering was the first to take a scientific approach when studying their properties. He worked with dried preparations of foxglove leaves and infusions, allowing more precise dosing than the concoctions traditionally used. His famous work *An Account of the Foxglove and some of its Medicinal Uses* summarized a decade of research and 163 case histories. In it, Withering warned that digitalis, the active component of the foxglove, would not work in all cases of dropsy and that it could have toxic effects.

"Time will fix the real value upon this discovery."
William Withering, speculating on the potential of digitalis

Digitalis became something of a panacea, being very widely prescribed throughout the 19th century. Modern research has shown that the drug is a cardiac glycoside—a compound that can be used, with caution, to treat heart failure. It is still prescribed today, on occasion, although it has been superseded by less toxic drugs.

Another of Withering's interests was the influence of climate on health. He, himself, had a weak chest and traveled often to Portugal in the hope that the hot dry climate there would do him some good. He was elected a foreign member of the Royal Academy of Sciences in Lisbon. It is likely Withering had tuberculosis and that this is what led to his death at the age of 58.

William Morton

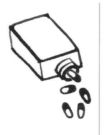

On October 16, 1846, a young printer, Gilbert Abbott, became the first person to undergo general anesthesia during an operation. With William Morton as the anesthetist, surgeon John Warren, of the Massachusetts General Hospital, carried out the 25-minute operation in which he removed a tumor from under Abbott's jaw. Using a hastily devised glass inhaler to administer ether vapor from a sea sponge soaked in the volatile liquid, Morton's work in solving the problem of pain relief was unrivaled.

Born: 1819, Charlton, Massachusetts
Importance: developed the use of ether as an anesthetic in dentistry and surgery
Died: 1868, New York, New York

Morton studied at the College of Dental Surgery in Baltimore, graduating in 1842. He then entered practice with Horace Wells. At the time, a number of dentists and surgeons were beginning to experiment with new ways of relieving pain during surgery. Although sedatives and analgesics such as opium and alcohol had long been known, it was not easy to operate on a patient in a stupor. The alternative was to operate without pain relief, which was inhumane and forced the surgeon to operate as quickly as possible. Thus, lack of controllable pain relief was a major barrier to the development of surgical technique.

The first attempts at anesthesia came from Thomas Beddoes and the chemist Humphry Davy, working in England. Davy noted how inhaling nitrous oxide dulled the pain of his erupting wisdom teeth, and produced a giddy feeling. Davy wrote, "As nitrous oxide in its extensive operation appears capable of destroying pain, it may probably be used with advantage during surgical operations."

In 1844, Wells began to use nitrous oxide for dental extraction and, the following year, he and Morton tried it out for minor surgery at the Massachusetts General Hospital. Nitrous oxide

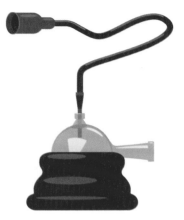

Left: William Morton manufactured inhalers for adminstering ether, a volatile liquid which he first saw used as a local anaesthetic by a chemistry professor at Harvard.

turned out not to be an ideal anesthetic, as it did not provide sufficient pain relief, and Wells was ridiculed for his efforts.

Meanwhile, Morton began to experiment with inhaled ether as a general anesthetic, which produces loss of consciousness, while a local anesthetic only produces loss of sensation (the term anesthesia comes from the Greek for "lack of feeling"). Morton started using ether in dental extractions and convinced John Warren to try it for the operation on Abbott.

News of Morton's innovation spread across America and to Europe. He started to manufacture the glass inhalers he used to administer the ether but would not reveal the details of his procedure because he wanted to patent it. A fight then broke out between Morton and Wells over who had invented anesthesia. With the dental practice failing, Morton was forced to abandon his career and took up farming in 1850. Meanwhile, the patent issue was never really settled.

In 1847, James Simpson in England introduced chloroform for anesthesia and this soon supplanted ether. Chloroform was widely used, although it is quite toxic, up until the 20th century. By then, the growing chemical industry was able to manufacture safer, nonflammable anesthetics. Today, anesthesia is a sophisticated medical speciality with the level of unconsciousness being very carefully controlled.

Pharmacologists

Homeopathy

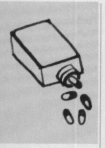

Homeopathy is a well-established system of alternative medicine. Despite experimental results that lend support to its claims, it is frequently ridiculed by the medical and scientific establishment. This is not surprising, since it has been said that, should homeopathic principles be demonstrated experimentally, the laws of physics would have to be rewritten. Homeopathy nevertheless continues to flourish, with thousands of registered homeopaths and pharmacies selling homeopathic remedies throughout the world.

Homeopathy was founded by Dr. Samuel Hahnemann (1755–1843), a German physician who felt dissatisfaction with the medical practices of his time, such as the excessive use of bloodletting, which he thought weakened the patient without any obvious benefit. He gave away his medical practice in 1790, 11 years after qualifying, and devoted his life to the development of homeopathy instead.

At its simplest, homeopathy is an alternative form of pharmacy: "drugs" are prescribed with a view to curing illness and disease. In contrast to orthodox medicine, the drugs are derived almost exclusively from natural sources and only occasionally from synthetic compounds. Homeopathy has great faith in the ability of the body to heal itself, that it has a natural balance, and that disease is a disruption of these central, regulating energies. It therefore aims to achieve a "homeostasis of vital functions," and talks about the "inner physician." It sees the homeopath as someone attempting to assist this process.

The approach of homeopathy is holistic: Rather than seeing each named illness as a separate entity and trying to cure it, it considers the sick person to be a unique individual who needs to thalidomide tragedy saw around 10,000 babies born with the rare congenital deformity of shortened or missing limbs after their mothers took thalidomide for conditions such as influenza and insomnia during pregnancy. Never again would drugs be allowed onto the market without thorough preliminary safety testing and that meant more animal experimentation. Tests are now carried out on pregnant animals to see if the drug causes effects like thalidomide, and they are tested on rabbits, mice, or rats to see if they cause cancer or adverse effects on the skin or eyes.

The Animals Act introduced in the UK in 1986 requires researchers to prove the benefits in improving human health will outweigh any suffering caused to animals involved in testing. The Public Health Service Policy on Humane Care and Use of Laboratory Animals, introduced in 1985, covered research funded by public money. Now, private companies and large universities in the US have to be accredited for work on animals.

There is an increasing emphasis on what is known as the "Three Rs"—principles laid down by Rex Burch and William Russell in *The Principles of Humane Experimental Technique*, published in 1959. The Three Rs are reduction, refinement, and replacement. Reduction means trying to minimize the number of experiments by, for example, harmonizing regulations so that experiments on drug safety do not have to be repeated in different countries. Refinement means extracting more information from fewer animal experiments. And there are many possible replacements, from using cells, tissues, and even organ slices, to using computer models and human volunteers for tests.

One development worrying animal rights advocates is the recent increase in the use of transgenic animal models for experiments. These animals have been genetically modified to carry a human gene, yielding data more relevant to humans who have the disease for which the drug is being developed.

Pharmacologists

Carl Djerassi

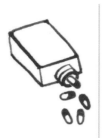

In 1951, Carl Djerassi achieved the first synthetic version of the female hormone, progesterone, producing a steroid called norethindrone. This drug became the most widely used active ingredient of the contraceptive pill. Now used by around 100 million women worldwide, "the Pill" remains unsurpassed to this day as a reversible contraceptive.

Born: 1923, Vienna, Austria

Importance: made a major contribution to the development of oral contraceptives, synthesizing one of the original versions of the Pill

Born into a Jewish family, Djerassi fled the Nazi regime with his mother, landing in New York in 1939. He studied chemistry at Kenyon College, Ohio, graduating in 1942. In 1949 he became Associate Director of Chemical Research at Syntex in Mexico City, where he carried out his groundbreaking work on the contraceptive pill.

Research had already shown that progesterone could stop ovulation in rabbits. However, natural progesterone is destroyed by the digestive system if taken orally, and so Djerassi's team set about developing the synthetic version, norethindrone. Both norethindrone and progesterone belong to a class of complex molecules known as steroids, and Djerassi had great expertise in the synthesis of steroids.

In 1950, Gregory Pincus, at the Worcester Foundation for Experimental Biology in Massachusetts, was asked by the Planned Parenthood Foundation to work on a new type of contraceptive, as people were dependent on on barrier methods, such as the diaphragm and the condom, which were not fully effective. It had to be something harmless, reliable, simple, practical, and acceptable to both husband and wife.

Djerassi sent some norethindrone to Pincus, who carried out animal studies with this and a related compound, norethynodrel.

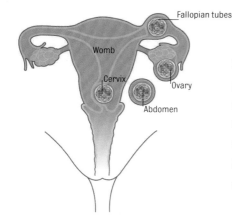

Left: Abulcasis was the first person to describe ectopic pregnancy, where fertilization of the egg occurs outside the womb, either, most commonly, in the Fallopian tubes, or in the cervix, ovary or abdomen.

laxatives, emetics, and appropriate dosages. He also discussed tablet-making, filtering, distillation, sublimation, and other drug-preparation techniques, and was the first to describe ectopic pregnancy, in 963. In the 12th century, *At-Tasrif* was translated into Latin by Gerard of Cremona and was used as a text in European medical training, alongside Avicenna's writings (see page 20), as late as the 17th century.

Albucasis is perhaps most famous for his writings on surgery, describing many surgical instruments, several of which he seems to have invented himself. Among 200 or so drawings, there are examples of catheters, tongue depressors, scalpels, curettes, and various instruments for obstetrics and extracting teeth. He talked about wound treatment, cauterizing to stop bleeding, bloodletting, and midwifery. He also mentioned the removal of cataracts from eyes and even breast reduction. He used catgut for internal stitching and forceps for extracting a dead fetus from its mother's body.

It appears that Albucasis treated many accident and injury cases in his practice, because his writings cover how to deal with fractures of the limbs and nose and how to treat a dislocated shoulder. A method of tying blood vessels often attributed to Ambroise Paré, the 16th-century French surgeon, was in fact first described by Abulcasis.

Practitioners

Thomas Sydenham

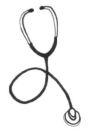

Thomas Sydenham reintroduced many of the principles of Hippocrates into English medicine. He did not favor any particular theory but tried to promote the power of observation and believed that the physician's experiences at the bedside were as important as a thorough knowledge of anatomy and physiology. He held views on disease that were surprisingly modern and largely in keeping with the opinions of doctors today.

Born: 1624, Wynford Eagle, England
Importance: known as the English Hippocrates, taught the power of careful observation in medicine; introduced several new remedies and treatments
Died: 1689, London, England

Sydenham's medical education was interrupted by military service in the English Civil War (1642–1651), where he took the side of the Parliamentarians. He graduated in medicine from Oxford in 1648 and did further studies in Montpelier, France. He subsequently obtained a license to practice from the Royal College of Physicians, in 1663, and worked as a doctor in Westminster. In London, he became friendly with the chemist Robert Boyle and the philosopher John Locke.

In keeping with his theories on observation, Sydenham believed in giving very precise descriptions of symptoms of diseases and their natural history. He was the first to diagnose scarlet fever and he wrote thorough accounts of gout, malaria, hysteria, and many other conditions. Doctors should, he argued, look for specific diseases and their corresponding causes. He believed that acute diseases, involving fever or inflammation, were the body's attempts to throw off malign influences—a concept that was a precursor to the germ theory of disease (see page 60). Chronic diseases, on the other hand, were an imbalance of the body's "humors" brought about by poor diet or some other lifestyle factor—an opinion which 21st century doctors would be in broad agreement with.

Sydenham's patients often got better because of the way he treated them. "I have the happiness of curing my patients," he said in a letter to Robert Boyle. He introduced iron for the treatment of anemia and used cinchona bark, a source of quinine, for malaria. He also believed in laudanum (a tincture of opium) for the treatment of severe pain. Unlike many physicians of this era, he did not rely overmuch on bloodletting, although he did use it on occasion.

Sydenham was one of the first physicians to study epidemiology—the causes and patterns of disease. He had experience of the Great Plague and of smallpox. He discussed the factors that might contribute to outbreaks of infectious diseases such as the season of the year and the nature of the weather. He is, perhaps, most famous for his approach to the treatment of fever. Most physicians believed patients should "sweat it out" and tried to increase a patient's temperature further by covering him or her with blankets. Sydenham argued for plenty of cool fluids and adequate ventilation.

Owing to his success as a physician, and his sound ideas, Sydenham became known as the "English Hippocrates" and also as the "Father of English Medicine." His fame spread after his death and he was often mentioned by medical teachers in Europe—although he was not without critics in his lifetime. He wrote a book on fevers in 1666, and followed it with volumes on other diseases. He eventually produced a comprehensive medical text, which became a classic. However, the disease named after him—Sydenham's chorea, an infectious disease of the nervous system characterized by jerky movements—occupies only a couple of small paragraphs in his book.

Percivall Pott

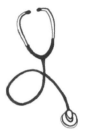

Percivall Pott was, in his day, Britain's leading surgeon, attracting large audiences to his lectures and running a private practice with prestigious patients including writer Samuel Johnson and painter Thomas Gainsborough. Determined to raise the rough-and-ready status of surgery to that of a respected medical profession, Pott advocated detailed observation, thorough practical training, and concern for the patient. The fact that he was successful in his aim is testimony to his consummate skill as a surgeon and the detailed studies that he wrote on a number of medical subjects.

Born: 1714, London, England
Importance: leading surgeon, who developed new operating techniques and did much to raise the status of his profession
Died: 1788, London, England

Pott became an apprentice surgeon at St. Bartholomew's Hospital, in London, in 1729. He studied under Edward Nourse and carried out duties such as preparing dissections for anatomy and surgery lectures. Even at this young age, his skill was apparent. He rose rapidly up the ranks at Barts, becoming a full surgeon in 1749. The Barber-Surgeons' Company, from which Pott soon acquired a diploma, became the Company of Surgeons in 1745 (the forerunner to the modern Royal College of Surgeons). Pott was a great advocate of surgery as a part of the medical profession, not just a practice in which a diseased part of the body was "sawed off." In 1753, Pott and William Hunter, the brother of John Hunter (see page 102), were appointed lecturers in anatomy to the Company, with Pott subsequently becoming examiner. He took up the position of Master of the Company in 1765.

In 1756 Pott was thrown from a horse and suffered a compound fracture of the femur. Normally the only remedy would have been immediate amputation, which was also life threatening.

Nourse advised against this, and Pott's leg healed successfully after the fracture was splinted. He later wrote an influential treatise on fractures. Pott also wrote detailed studies on a number of other conditions, including anal fistula, head wounds, and cancer.

John Hunter became one of Pott's pupils and his work on anatomy and pathology helped advance surgical knowledge. Pott was elected a member of the Royal Society, because of his writings on operations and diseases, and he also succeeded Nourse as senior surgeon at Barts, in 1765. His name lives on in two medical conditions: Pott's disease is described in his research into palsy, where he found a relationship between spinal curvature (now known to be a form of tuberculosis) and paralysis of the lower limbs; while Pott's fracture is a fracture dislocation of the ankle.

"Many and great are the improvements which the chirurgical art has received in the last 50 years, and many thanks are due to those who contributed to them; but when we reflect how much still remains to be done, it should rather excite our industry rather than inflame our vanity."

Percivall Pott

Pott famously spotted the link between exposure to soot—an occupational hazard for chimney sweeps—and an increased risk of cancer of the scrotum. This was the first time an occupational cause for cancer had been identified and also the first documented case of an environmental carcinogen. Pott's work led to the introduction of the Chimney Sweepers Act in 1788, which recognized the hazard posed to health by soot and made it illegal to employ children younger than eight as chimney sweeps.

John Hunter

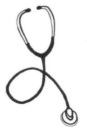

With a deep-rooted fascination for anatomy, surgeon John Hunter made a number of significant discoveries about the workings of the human body through his many animal experiments and human dissections. Becoming one of London's most active medical researchers in the second half of the eighteenth century, he gave a total of 27 papers to the Royal Society in the last 30 to 40 years of his life, on subjects as diverse as the sense of smell, digestion, the growth of bones, and animal behavior.

Born: 1728, Long Calderwood, Scotland

Importance: leading comparative anatomist, pathologist, and surgeon who amassed a large collection of specimens to support his theories of disease

Died: 1793, London, England

Hunter traveled to London in 1748 to train with his elder brother, the distinguished anatomist William Hunter. Later he also trained in surgery at Chelsea and St. Bartholomew's Hospitals. Hunter was fascinated by anatomy and carried out many animal experiments. He became skilled in anatomy, working on corpses provided by the "resurrectionists," who stole them from graveyards for a price. He also worked as an army surgeon in the Seven Years War (1756–1763).

Returning to London after the war, Hunter found it hard to find a surgical position, despite his experience, so he began working with the London dentist James Spence. Despite the lowly status given to dentistry at the time, Hunter continued to make valuable discoveries. He produced his first major publication, *A Treatise on the Natural History of the Human Teeth*, in 1771. It was the first scientific text on dentistry to be produced in English.

Hunter discussed teeth in the context of his detailed researches on the anatomy of muscles and bones of the jaw and face. He explained how mastication occurred by the action of various muscle groups. He was also interested in how teeth

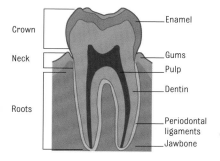

Crown

Neck

Roots

Enamel

Gums

Pulp

Dentin

Periodontal
ligaments

Jawbone

Left: John Hunter was one of the first people to study the anatomy of teeth in a scientific manner, including the structure of the tooth and the muscles and bones of the jaw. This had a great impact on both medicine and dentistry.

develop both in the fetus and the child. His interest in comparative anatomy led him to study the differences between carnivores and herbivores. His treatise gave clinical advice to dentists on how "calcareous deposits" could cause gum disease and on how best to extract teeth. He was also interested in the possible transplantation of teeth: he carried out a famous experiment in which he transplanted a tooth into the comb of a cockerel.

Hunter finally obtained a post as surgeon at St. George's Hospital, London, and became physician to King George III in 1778. This pleased him because it gave him access to the king's menagerie for experiments. His wide scientific and medical interests were reflected in his famous collection of thousands of human and animal specimens. When one of the royal elephants died, George III donated its body to Hunter's collection. It was purchased by the government in 1799, after Hunter's death, and now resides on the premises of the Royal College of Surgeons in London.

Among Hunter's most famous books was *A Treatise on the Venereal Diseases*, in which he argued (wrongly) that gonorrhea and syphilis were the same disease. He may even have tried to prove this by injecting himself with syphilis in order to study the course of the disease. This experiment may have played a role in his death, although he also suffered from angina for many years.

Practitioners

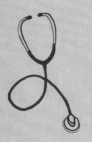

Transplantation

The idea of repairing and renewing damaged parts of the body—known in recent years as regenerative medicine—has its origins in the early days of organ transplantation. Successful transplantation of kidneys between identical twins first occurred in 1954 and, in 1962, between unrelated donors and recipients. In the 1954 operation, performed by Joseph Murray and his team at Peter Bent Brigham Hospital, Boston, a kidney was transplanted from eight-year-old Ronald Herrick into his twin Richard, who lived for another eight years. The work earned Murray a Nobel Prize for Physiology of Medicine in 1990.

The next landmark was the transplant of a single lung, in 1963, by James Hardy of the University of Mississippi, but his patient died within a few days. In 1967 Thomas Starzl carried out the first successful liver transplant (see page 120). But the operation that really hit the headlines was Christiaan Barnard's transplant of a human heart in the same year in Cape Town. Here, a man with advanced heart failure received the heart of a young girl who had died in a road accident.

The first combined heart, liver, and kidney transplant was carried out in Pittsburgh in 1989, on a young woman who survived for four months. In recent years, many other parts of the body have been transplanted for the first time—the larynx, the womb, the penis and even, in 2005, the face. The outcome for the patients in these "firsts" varies—some are still alive, others did not survive for long. However, they have all contributed more than anyone to making transplantation a life-saving operation.

Nor would these operations have been possible without a great deal of pioneering research into the immune system. In the 1940s, British scientist Peter Medawar showed that animal embryos exposed to foreign tissues do not reject them and concluded that rejection is based on immunologic factors. Meanwhile, Frank McFarlane Burnet, of the University of Melbourne, suggested the body's immune cells learn early on to accept tissues that are present as part of the body but will later reject any new material. Together this research formed the discovery of acquired immunological tolerance, which is the basis of modern immunosuppressant therapy regimes. The two won the 1960 Nobel Prize for Physiology or Medicine for their work.

The drug cyclosporin, derived from a soil fungus, was introduced in the 1980s to help patients avoid rejecting their new organs. In 1990, tacrolimus, related to cyclosporin but about 100 times more potent, was launched. Meanwhile, surgical techniques have been improved to the extent that living donors can be operated on safely. Once reserved for the most desperately ill patients, an organ transplant is now almost a routine procedure for many.

There is, however, a serious gap between supply and demand in organ transplantation. This is partly due to aging populations leading to increases in chronic diseases for which an organ transplant is a feasible treatment option (kidney failure and congestive heart failure), as well as the burden of hepatitis C, a blood-borne viral infection, which is now a leading indication for liver transplantation. However, changes in legislation on donor cards and improved coordination are helping to boost the number of donors. There has also been an increase in the use of living donors and organs from older cadavers. But the gap remains, and is likely to do so for the foreseeable future. Although there have been advances in the science of xenotransplantation (the use of genetically modified organs from animals) and in mechanical assist devices (such as artificial hearts) they are not likely to make a major contribution to the ongoing and increasing need.

Practitioners

Joseph Lister

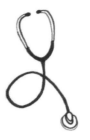

Taking his lead from Louis Pasteur's work on microbiology (see page 54), Joseph Lister investigated the problem of post-surgery wound infection, which was often fatal. He reasoned the air in the operating theater must be contaminated with infection-causing germs. In an attempt to limit the wound's contact with air, Lister introduced carbolic acid into wound management, bringing about the use of an antiseptic.

Born: 1827, Upton, England
Importance: pioneered use of antisepsis in surgery
Died: 1912, Walmer, England

Lister entered University College London in 1844, where he was greatly influenced by the leading physiologist William Sharpey and the surgeon Thomas Wharton Jones, both expert microscopists. Lister received awards for his work in pathology, anatomy, and surgery. He graduated in 1852 and became a Fellow of the Royal College of Surgeons.

Lister moved to Edinburgh Royal Infirmary, where he worked with James Syme, a friend of Sharpey's, learning more about surgery and carrying out experiments on inflammation and blood clotting. In 1857, he presented a paper to the Royal Society entitled "The Early Stages of Inflammation." In 1860, Lister became Professor of Surgery at Glasgow University and, the following year, took up a post as surgeon at Glasgow Royal Infirmary.

As a medical student, in 1846, Lister had witnessed England's first-ever operation carried out under anesthesia. Although the use of anesthesia had greatly expanded the range of operations carried out, the death rate after surgery was as high as 40 percent, because patients often succumbed to wound infections and sepsis. It was widely believed that sepsis occurred as a result of a reaction between moist exposed tissue and air.

Lister developed his germ theory (see page 60) in 1865, having been introduced to Louis Pasteur's work by chemistry professor Thomas Anderson. He decided to kill any germs in the air of the operating theater and also to exclude air from the surgical wound. He introduced the antiseptic, carbolic acid, into the wound during an operation on a compound fracture of the leg of an 11-year-old boy, spraying the acid on the wound and covering it with clean lint soaked in the antiseptic. The boy made a complete recovery, free of sepsis. In 1867, Lister was able to claim there had not been a single case of sepsis on his wards for nine months.

Sepsis: A condition in which bacteria, and maybe bacterial toxins, enter the bloodstream, possibly leading to shock, organ failure, and death.

Lister published a set of papers in the *British Medical Journal*, arguing for the adoption of his antiseptic methods. His claims were controversial, even though he cited Pasteur and presented sound scientific arguments for his work. In fact, other surgeons were working on preventing sepsis using different antiseptics, while others argued simple cleanliness would suffice. Lister was also in favor of strict hygiene, insisting on immersing surgical instruments in carbolic acid to prevent the spread of infection; later he used steam sterilization instead, following the suggestion of microbiologist Robert Koch (see page 56).

Lister returned to London in 1877 and became professor of surgery at Kings College. He and his followers were responsible for many improvements in surgery in the late 19th century. He also introduced absorbable stitches, new dressings, and wound drainage, as well as pioneering the radical mastectomy and wiring of fractured patellae. In 1887 he was made a baron in recognition of his work. He was one of the founders of the British Institute of Preventive Medicine, which was renamed the Lister Institute in his honor, in 1903.

Florence Nightingale

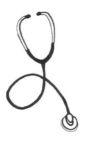

For many, the image of Florence Nightingale is a sentimental one—the "lady with the lamp," comforting the sick. She was also a superb organizer and advocate who turned nursing into a respectable profession for young, intelligent women and promoted it as a true vocation in life. She was a huge inspiration to others: by the end of the 19th century, so fierce was the competition in nursing that it was hard for young women to find a training place.

Born: 1829, Florence, Italy
Importance: a social reformer who helped establish nursing as a modern, secular profession
Died: 1910, London, England

Florence Nightingale fought her parents' opposition to her becoming a nurse for many years, eventually traveling to Pastor Theodore Fliedner's Deaconesses Institute, a religious training school for nurses in Kaiserwerth, Germany, one of the first training centers of its kind. She spent three months there and also studied with the Sisters of Mercy in Paris. She returned to England in 1853 and became superintendent of the Hospital for Invalid Gentlewomen.

The Crimean War broke out in 1853 and, through her friendship with the Secretary of War, Sidney Herbert, Nightingale was invited to travel to Scutari, in Turkey, where reports of deplorable conditions at the British military hospitals had filtered back to England through the reports written by *The Times* journalist W. N. Russell. Nightingale and her party of 38 nurses found around 1,000 wounded soldiers living in squalor with very limited food supplies. She set about cleaning up and reorganizing the hospital, applying strict standards of hygiene and insisting on adequate ventilation. After six months the death rate among the soldiers had come down from 42 percent to just 2 percent.

Nightingale returned to England a heroine at the end of the war. She promoted further reforms in both domestic and military nursing. A public fund raised over $200,000 to establish the Nightingale School and Home for Nurses, which opened in St. Thomas Hospital, London, in 1860. Around this time she published the manual *Notes on Nursing*, which laid out her principles.

She also campaigned for better conditions in military hospitals. A Royal Commission introduced many of her recommendations including a radical reform of sanitary conditions in barracks and the establishment of an army medical school. Nightingale then retired from public life, confined to her bed with a mystery illness, although she continued to issue reports and recommendations.

> "It may seem a strange principle to enunciate as the very first requirement in a hospital that it should do the sick no harm."
>
> Florence Nightingale

Before Florence Nightingale, nursing had been a job associated with lower class, disreputable women or with religious orders. Her location of a training school within a hospital is significant, as she believed that doctors and nurses should work side by side (although it was not an equal partnership, with nurses deferring to doctors). The Nightingale system of strict discipline, organization, and hygiene soon spread, with schools being established in Australia, New Zealand, and Canada. Nightingale was not a scientist. Her passion for hygiene was more related to her strong religious beliefs than a wish to avoid germs, as she did not believe in germ theory (see page 60). Her work also led Henri Dunant to found the Red Cross in 1854, which helped promote nursing training in less developed countries. In 1908, Florence Nightingale became the first woman ever to be awarded the Order of Merit.

William Osler

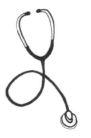

For his many talents, William Osler is often regarded as the father of modern medicine. He was the first physician to consider the patient to be as important as the disease and also carried out important scientific and clinical work, with a number of diseases and symptoms named after him.

Born: 1849, Ontario, Canada
Importance: developed medical education in the US and England, with his combination of bedside manner and sound science
Died: 1919, Oxford, England

Osler studied medicine in Toronto, then moved to McGill University in Montreal, graduating from there in 1872. He subsequently made a tour of various European medical institutions, before becoming a professor at McGill. He obtained a post as a physician at Montreal General Hospital in 1878, before taking up a chair of medicine at the University of Pennsylvania. He is perhaps best known for his long connection with Johns Hopkins University, a world-renowned medical institution, where he was a founding professor.

Osler's approach to the training of doctors was to make sure they were both compassionate and scientific in their work. He insisted his students got plenty of "hands-on" experience with patients and learned how to observe and communicate with them. His book *Theory and Practices of Medicine*, published in 1892, became a classic, with 20 editions published in total (the last being in 2001).

> "The good physician treats the disease, but the great physician treats the patient who has the disease."
>
> William Osler

After 15 years at Johns Hopkins, Osler moved to England to become Regius Professor of Medicine at the University of Oxford. He expanded the preclinical department to ensure students had a

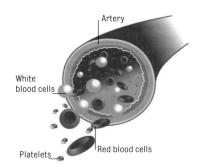

White
blood cells

Artery

Platelets

Red blood cells

Left: William Osler was the first physician to identify platelets as a separate component of blood. Platelets are small, clear components of blood that adhere together to help blood clot.

firm grounding in science. He founded the Association of Physicians of Great Britain and Northern Ireland and the *Quarterly Journal of Medicine*. He was also able to devote more time to long-standing interests in history, literature, and the classics. Osler became a baronet for his services to medicine in the Coronation Honors List of 1911.

Osler was the first physician to study platelets, which he wrote about in 1873. Three diseases discovered in the early years of the 20th century were named after him: Osler-Rendu-Weber disease (a disease of the blood vessels), Vasquez-Osler's disease (a blood disease), and Osler's nodes (an infection of the membrane covering the heart). A number of signs and symptoms are also named after him, such as Osler's sign, which is an artificially high blood pressure reading.

Osler was a prolific writer and a popular public speaker. Many of his quotes have passed into medical folklore, such as his saying that "it is much more important to know what sort of patient has a disease than what sort of disease a patient has." He was also a collector of medical books and left his library to McGill University, where it formed the basis of the Osler Library of the History of Medicine, opened in 1929. Osler and his wife died in the great flu pandemic of 1919. His obituary in *The Lancet* described him as "the greatest personality in the medical world."

Practitioners

Sigmund Freud

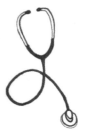

Sigmund Freud developed a theory of psychoanalysis that turned him into a celebrated international figure. Several of his concepts have entered mainstream language—the "Freudian slip"—for example. He is also the father of a number of innovative approaches to therapy, including the use of free association and dream interpretation.

Born: 1856, Freiberg, Austria
Importance: founder of the school of thought known as psychoanalysis
Died: 1939, London, England

Freud began his academic career as a medical student in Vienna, graduating in 1881. After period of study in Paris with the great French neurologist Jean Martin Charcot, Freud decided to devote himself to psychology. His interest in medical matters continued, however; at various times he was considered an authority on the cerebral palsies of children, produced publications on the anatomy and physiology of the nervous system, an important monograph on aphasia, and the first enquiry into the potential medical uses of cocaine.

Psychoanalysis began as an approach to treatment, but developed into a theory of the mind in general. Initially controversial, Freud's theories gained global renown. Some have criticized his work for reflecting too much of his own personal psychology, therefore lacking the general validity he assumed. This may be why he found it hard to retain his followers: Carl Jung, Alfred Adler, Otto Rank, and Wilhelm Reich all left him, going on to develop their own distinct psychological theories.

Of Freud's concepts, the best known today include the Freudian slip (an unintentional mistake or slip of the tongue that reveals a truth that the conscious mind is trying to conceal) and the Oedipus complex (the idea that a boy wants to have sexual relations with his mother, seeing the father as a rival and obstacle). Then there is the idea of ego, id, and superego (the tripartite division of the psyche: the ego is the conscious part striving to adapt, to be civilized; the id is primitive, with instinctual desires; and the superego has a critical and moralizing function, an inner parent as it were).

Freud's innovations were several. He pioneered the use of free association as a technique for the scientific examination of the human mind. He is famous for his recognition of the role of transference in the therapeutic relationship. He was also one of the first to note that hysteria was the product of a physical trauma that had been forgotten by the patient.

Other noteworthy aspects of Freudian theory include his use of dream interpretation as a therapeutic tool. He described dreams as the "royal road to the unconscious." He believed dreams represented the disguised fulfilment of unconscious wishes, predominantly sexual, and that their bizarre nature was due to a censoring function, which attempts to prevent them from being understood by the conscious ego. He also believed that sexuality was the main motivational force in human personality.

"The concept of the unconscious has long been knocking at the gates of psychology and asking to be let in. Philosophy and literature have often toyed with it, but science could find no use for it."

Sigmund Freud

Freud was a prolific writer. Perhaps his most famous book, and the most important in his own estimation, is *The Interpretation of Dreams*. Also notable is *The Psychopathology of Everyday Life*—the source of the idea of the Freudian slip—which is significant because in it Freud applied his theories to the general public, not just to the neurotic.

Emil Kraepelin

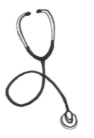

Emil Kraepelin is most famous for his work on psychosis and the distinction he made between schizophrenia and manic depression. He also described paranoia. He firmly believed that mental illnesses were biological or genetic and not a sign of moral weakness. The biological view he presented now dominates modern psychiatry.

Born: 1856, Neustrelitz, Germany
Importance: devised a classification of mental illnesses and was the first to distinguish between schizophrenia and bipolar disorder
Died: 1926, Munich, Germany

Kraepelin studied medicine at Leipzig and Würzburg, receiving his medical degree in 1878. In Leipzig he came under the influence of the great experimental psychologist Wilhelm Wundt and wrote a prize-winning essay entitled "The influence of acute illness in the causation of mental disorders."

Kraepelin completed a PhD at the University of Munich with a thesis on the role of psychology in psychiatry. He returned to Leipzig and carried out research on psychopharmacology with Wundt, also practicing neurology. In 1883, he published his influential *Compendium of Psychiatry*, in which he argued that psychiatry should be considered a branch of medical science. He was the first to be interested in the role of brain pathology in mental illness, basing his theories on clinical and experimental observations.

Kraepelin's name for schizophrenia was "dementia praecox" (premature dementia). This later proved to be a misnomer, as schizophrenia is not a form of dementia. Kraepelin called it dementia because he had noted that schizophrenia has a deteriorating course. Manic depression, in contrast, has a relapsing-remitting pattern, with patients being symptom-free between episodes of either mania or depression. In a series of lectures, published in 1901, Kraepelin pointed out that the schizophrenic could be intelligent but withdrawn into a world of his own and lost touch with reality. He referred to the condition as "atrophy of emotions" and "vitiation of the will," both good descriptions of the so-called negative symptoms of schizophrenia.

In 1904, Kraepelin became director of a new psychiatric clinic in Munich, which became a renowned center for the teaching of psychiatry. He rejected Freud's psychoanalytic theories (see page 112) and continued to develop his work on the biological basis of mental illness. In his experiments, he studied the nature of sleep and the impact on intoxicants, such as alcohol and morphine, on the central nervous system.

Kraepelin was a social reformer, crusading against alcohol, capital punishment, and indefinite prison sentences. He also established the German Institute of Psychiatric Research.

Despite his work being obscured by Freud for much of the 20th century, interest in Kraeplin's work has been revived in recent years. His classifications of mental illness have influenced American Psychiatric Association's DSM-IV system and the ICD system of the World Health Organization (WHO). The biological view, and the use of psychopharmacology foreshadowed by his work, now dominate modern psychiatry. Progress in understanding the brain and techniques like brain imaging have also revealed the truth of his predictions on the role of brain pathology in mental disease.

> "[Sexual excitability] is increased and leads to hasty engagements, marriages by the newspaper, improper love-adventures, conspicuous behavior, fondness for dress, on the other hand to jealousy and matrimonial discord."
>
> Emil Kraeplin, on mania

Harvey Cushing

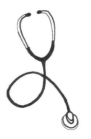

The first physician to measure blood pressure, Harvey Cushing is best known for his unrivaled contribution to brain surgery. Thanks to a number of innovative techniques introduced by him, the death rate from brain surgery fell from 90 percent to just 10 percent. During his career Cushing removed over 2,000 brain tumors. He was a talented artist and his drawings of the brains on which he operated became a central part of his surgical reports.

Born: 1869, Cleveland, Ohio
Importance: pioneering brain surgeon, who also carried out significant research on blood pressure and the pituitary gland
Died: 1939, New Haven, Connecticut

The son of a physician, Cushing studied medicine at Yale and Harvard universities, graduating in 1895. He then studied surgery at Johns Hopkins University under the famous surgeon William Halsted and showed great surgical skill. He researched the effects on intracranial pressure, experimenting on dogs, and applied his findings to the diagnosis, localization, and removal of intracranial tumors in humans.

Until the 20th century, the brain was the only part of the body that was not regularly operated on, as cutting into the brain invariably led to massive blood loss, on severance of the intricate network of blood vessels serving the brain. The death rate from brain surgery was as high as 90 percent.

Cushing changed that, devising clips and clamps to pinch off bleeding blood vessels during an operation. He used X-rays to diagnose tumors and performed craniotomies—cutting of the skull to get at the brain—using only a local anesthetic (the brain is not sensitive to pain). Patients began to survive previously fatal brain tumors, and deaths fell to 10 percent.

Cushing became Professor of Surgery at Harvard University in 1912, teaching his new neurosurgical techniques. One of his

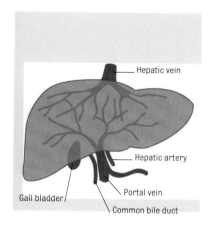

Hepatic vein

Hepatic artery

Portal vein

Gall bladder

Common bile duct

Left: Starzl's pioneering work on liver transplants showed that a full liver transplant required taking not only the liver, but also the gall bladder, severing and reattaching the hepatic vein, hepatic artery, portal vein, and common bile duct.

operation was unsuccessful, due to uncontrolled bleeding, and Starzl was criticized. Undeterred, he carried out a second liver transplant a few weeks later on a man with liver cancer. To avert bleeding, he gave the patient large amounts of an anti-clotting drug. The operation appeared to work, but the man died three weeks later from complications owing to blood clotting.

Over the next few years, Starzl carried out further work on immune suppression and also looked at tissue-matching techniques. In 1967, he attempted his third liver transplant, and the patient survived. In the same year, Christiaan Barnard, working in Cape Town, carried out the first successful human heart transplant. By the late 1970s, liver transplantation had improved so much that the survival rate had risen to 40 percent.

Starzl was responsible for the first intestine, liver, pancreas, and spleen transplant, in 1983, and the first heart and liver transplant, in 1984. He also did important work on the preservation and procurement of organs and, with British transplant pioneer Sir Roy Calne, carried out groundbreaking work on immuno-suppressant drugs that have helped make transplantation an almost routine procedure. Once considered as a procedure of last resort, for whom only the desperately sick were considered, organ transplantation is now offered to a wider range of patients (see page 104).

Patrick Steptoe

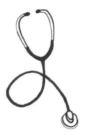

In 1976 29-year-old patient Lesley Brown was referred to Patrick Steptoe. Brown had severely damaged Fallopian tubes and she and her husband, John, had been trying to have a baby for 10 years. On November 10, 1977, Steptoe took an egg from Brown and fertilized it in the laboratory. When the embryo reached the eight-cell stage, after two and a half days, Steptoe and his colleague Robert Edwards implanted it. Baby Louise Brown was born on July 25, 1978—the world's first successful in vitro baby.

Born: 1913, Oxford, England
Importance: pioneered in-vitro fertilization (IVF) to help infertile couples have children
Died: 1988, Canterbury, England

Patrick Steptoe studied at King's College London, and St. George's Hospital Medical School at the University of London, becoming a member of the Royal College of Surgeons in 1939. After studying obstetrics and gynecology in Manchester, he took up a position at Oldham General Hospital in 1951. He became interested in methods of sterilization and in the problem of infertility.

Steptoe promoted the use of laparoscopy, a technique in which an optical device is used to examine the inside of the abdomen through a minute incision. This was the forerunner of minimally invasive surgery, in which miniaturized instruments are inserted through an incision to carry out a range of procedures that would otherwise be done by open surgery.

"I am not a wizard or a Frankenstein. All I want to do is help women whose child-producing mechanism is slightly faulty."

Patrick Steptoe

In 1966 Steptoe teamed up with Robert Edwards, a physiologist at Cambridge University, who had achieved the fertilization of a human egg in the laboratory, helping women with blocked Fallopian tubes become pregnant. Meanwhile, Steptoe developed the use of laparoscopy to retrieve eggs from a woman's ovary. This set the scene for in vitro fertilization (IVF). The pair reasoned if eggs retrieved from the ovaries could then be fertilized in the laboratory (that is, "in vitro"—literally, in glass), the resulting embryo could then be implanted in the woman's uterus and a pregnancy could develop.

Although refused funding by the UK Medical Research Council, Steptoe and Edwards were able to continue work on IVF after the Ford Foundation in the United States provided the money needed.

In 1972, they carried out the first IVF, but the embryo did not implant in the uterus. In the next few years, some pregnancies did occur through IVF, but all miscarried in the first three months. They had their first success in 1976 with the IVF that led to Lesley Brown's pregacy. Although she developed toxemia during the last few weeks, meaning that a Cesarean section was needed, her baby was born without complication, weighing in at 5lb 12oz (2.5kg).

Steptoe's and Edward's achievement marked the beginning of assisted reproductive technology. Despite criticism from religious groups accusing them of "playing God," and ethical questions about what should happen to fertilized eggs that were not implanted, IVF offered new hope to infertile couples and Steptoe received thousands of letters from those wanting to try it. Steptoe and Edwards set up Bourn Hall Clinic near Cambridge to teach others the IVF procedure. Over three million babies have now been born by IVF around the world.

Toxemia: Also known as preeclampsia, toxemia of pregnancy is a condition marked by high blood pressure and fluid retention that may arise in the second half of pregnancy, potentially leading to full-blown eclampsia with seizures and a high risk of maternal and fetal mortality.

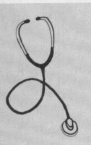

Euthanasia and Palliative Care

Increases in life expectancy during the 20th century led to an attitude of denial toward the natural processes of death and dying. Patients with cancer were often not told their diagnosis, and those dying in hospitals got no special treatment or support. Worse, painkilling drugs were often withheld in the false belief that a patient might become addicted. Advances in medicine often set up false expectations that there must always be a cure, and doctors often took the death of a patient as a personal failure.

The English nurse and physician Cicely Saunders set out to ease the physical and emotional suffering of the dying in the 1950s (see page 126). She first aimed to better understand the principles of pain control, so that powerful opioid drugs, like morphine, could be administered to prevent, rather than relieve, pain. Doses were carefully adjusted so the patient stayed pain free yet alert, enabling them to make the most of the time they had left. Effective pain control became the focus of palliative care—care that aims to support and comfort, rather than cure, and is applicable to patients with advanced, progressive diseases.

Saunders believed palliative care was best administered in a specialist setting. The hospice movement had already begun in France and Ireland in the late-19th century, but the first modern hospice was St. Joseph's Hospice in London, which opened in 1958 and pioneered developments in palliative pain control. Saunders opened her own, St. Christopher's Hospice, in 1967 and it soon became a center of excellence for caring for the terminally ill and training doctors and nurses in palliative care. The hospice movement later spread to the United States and beyond.

The principles of palliative care involve doing all that is needed to let patients live to their remaining physical and mental potential. They are encouraged to decide where they wish to end their days, be it at home or in a hospice setting, and given appropriate support to fulfill this choice. Family and friends are offered the support they need, both while their loved one is still alive and afterward, during the bereavement process. Palliative care has now become a part of mainstream medicine, with some hospice units located within hospitals. Attitudes have also changed. It is now viewed as unethical to withhold a terminal diagnosis from a patient, although the news needs to be broken gradually, if necessary, and with great sensitivity.

Lack of palliative care can lead some terminal patients to wish for euthanasia, or assisted suicide, in which someone, such as a doctor, helps them end their life. Although doctors are not obliged to actively treat someone when they have no hope of recovery, this is not the same as administering euthanasia (although the withdrawal of treatment may cause the patient's death).

Euthanasia is illegal in most countries. One argument against it is a religious one—that God alone has the right to decide when a life should end. Another is the "slippery slope" argument, that the criteria for euthanasia will be relaxed gradually, so that people who are a burden to themselves and others, rather than terminally ill, will be killed. Indeed, some sick or elderly people could feel pressured into agreeing to euthanasia, if it were legal, because they fear either their own suffering or becoming a burden to their family or even the state. At present euthanasia is only legal in Belgium and the Netherlands. Switzerland allows assisted suicide and does not view this as euthanasia. In Oregon, a physician is allowed to supply a lethal dose of medication to a patient, but euthanasia itself remains illegal.

Cicely Saunders

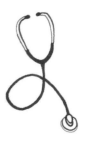

With a firm belief that everyone has the right to die pain free and with dignity, Cicely Saunders was the first doctor to devote her whole career to the care of the dying. Her work, now recognized as the beginning of palliative care (see page 124), earned her an international reputation and influenced the way in which many countries view terminal illness and death.

Born: 1918, Barnet, England
Importance: campaigned to relieve end-of-life physical and emotional suffering
Died: 2005, London, England

Saunders was brought up in a wealthy family and educated at Roedean, England's leading girls' boarding school. She went to Oxford to study, but left to train as a nurse. In 1948, she fell in love with a Polish patient, David Tasma, who was dying of cancer. He left her $2,000 in his will to found a hospice. She later trained in medicine at the age of 39, because she wanted to understand the best way of controlling terminal pain. She received her degree in 1957, and soon began research into pain control, working at St. Joseph Hospice in London, where nursing care was provided for the dying. She developed the idea of anticipating and preventing pain through the detailed understanding of the various analgesic drugs so the patient could receive effective doses that would leave them alert. Previously, powerful analgesics had often been withheld from patients in pain, for fear of their developing an addiction to the drugs.

St. Christopher's Hospice, the project begun with Tasma's bequest, was finally opened in southeast London in 1967, with Saunders as its director. Her work there focused on relieving physical and the associated emotional suffering. Although reliance on medicine remained—and still does—on the curative side, Saunders's work began to encourage many doctors in Europe and the United States to include this palliative element in their practice. A deeply religious woman, Saunders did not believe in euthanasia. This made it even more important for her patients to have quality of life right to the end.

In 1980, Saunders was made a Dame and married the artist Professor Marian Bohusz-Szyszko, who was to have a great influence on her life and work. She nursed him through a long illness before his death in St. Christopher's in 1995. In 1989, Saunders became one of only a few women in the United Kingdom to receive the Order of Merit. She herself died in St. Christopher's at the age of 87.

Today there are 7,000 to 8,000 palliative-care facilities in more than 100 countries around the world. They can be found in a number of settings—independent hospices offering community-based care and day care, in-patient facilities integrated into a hospital setting, and specialist teams who go out into the community offering their services.

> "You matter because you are you, and you matter to the last moment of your life."
>
> Cicely Saunders

There are many different aspects of the work of a hospice. Symptom control is key—whether it is pain relief or treatment of problems such as breathlessness. Complementary therapies, such as art therapy and aromatherapy, offer both physical and mental benefit to the patient. The ideas of palliative care are now firmly established, but their practice is not as widespread as they should be. Demand for palliative care will grow as the population ages, however. No matter how sophisticated the latest scientific advances, medicine will never be able to cure everything and people will always need end-of-life care.

Glossary

acupuncture System of Chinese medicine involving the insertion of fine needles at specific points on the body in order to affect the flow of energy and thereby improve health.

antigen Foreign substance that triggers the body's immune system.

aromatherapy Practice of using plant essential oils for healing.

circulatory system The system of the body responsible for circulating blood.

differential diagnosis Determining a disease or condition among several that share the same symptoms.

dissection Cutting into a body to determine what is inside.

homeopathy Treatment that uses small amounts of natural substances that would cause illness if used in large doses.

lesion Abnormality in tissue.

nucleotide A basic unit of DNA.

pandemic Outbreak of a disease that is far-reaching.

pathology Branch of science that studies the causes of disease.

pharmacogenetics The branch of genetics that looks at how an individual processes the drugs he or she is prescribed.

physiology Branch of science that studies the way organisms and their parts function.

pneumococci A bacteria associated with pneumonia.

posthumous Occurring after a person's death.

postulate A suggestion or theory for further study.

prophylactic Medicine or treatment intended to prevent disease.

sepsis Harmful toxins in the tissues of a body.

tuberculosis A disease affecting the body's tissue, particularly the lungs.

vivisection Animal experimentation.

vizier Muslim high official.

For More Information

American Association for the History of Medicine
509 N. 12th St
Box 980582
Richmond, VA 23298
(804) 828-9898
Website: http://www.histmed.org
The American Association for the History of Medicine (AAHM),
founded in 1925, is a professional association of historians,
physicians, nurses, archivists, curators, librarians, and others.
The AAHM promotes and encourages research, study, writing,
and interest in the history of medicine, including the history of
public health, dentistry, pharmacy, nursing and allied arts,
sciences, and professions.

American Association for the History of Nursing
10200 W. 44th Ave., Suite 304
Wheat Ridge, CO 80033
(303) 422-2685
Website: http://www.aahn.org
The American Association for the History of Nursing (AAHN) is
a professional organization open to everyone interested in the
history of nursing. Originally founded in 1978 as a historical
methodology group, the association was briefly named the
International History of Nursing Society. The purpose of the
Association is to foster the importance of history as relevant to
understanding the past, defining the present, and influencing the
future of nursing.

American Medical Association (AMA)
AMA Plaza
330 N. Wabash Ave.
Chicago, IL 60611-5885
(800) 621-8335
Website: http://www.ama-assn.org
The mission of the AMA is to promote the art and science of
medicine and the betterment of public health. Since 1847, the
American Medical Association has promoted scientific
advancement, improved public health, and invested in the
doctor and patient relationship.

Canadian Society for the History of Medicine
Brock University
500 Glenridge Ave.
St. Catharines, ON L2S 3A1
Canada
Website: http://www.cshm-schm.ca
The Canadian Society for the History of Medicine promotes the
study of the history of health and medicine. Since 1978, the
organization has held annual conferences in conjunction with
the Congress of the Social Sciences and Humanities.

U.S. National Library of Medicine
Reference and Web Services
National Library of Medicine
8600 Rockville Pike
Bethesda, MD 20894
(888) 346-3656
Website: http://www.nim.nih.gov
The National Library of Medicine (NLM) has been a center of
information innovation since its founding in 1836. The world's
largest biomedical library, NLM maintains and makes available
a vast print collection and produces electronic information
resources on a wide range of topics that are searched billions of
times each year by millions of people around the globe. It also
supports and conducts research, development, and training in
biomedical informatics and health information technology. In
addition, the Library coordinates a 6,000-member National
Network of Libraries of Medicine that promotes and provides
access to health information in communities across the United
States.

Websites

Because of the changing nature of Internet links, Rosen Publishing
has developed an online list of websites related to the subject of
this book. This site is updated regularly. Please use this link to
access the list:

http://www.rosenlinks.com/THINK/Med

For Further Reading

Anderson, Julie. *The Art of Medicine*. Chicago, IL: University of Chicago Press, 2012.

Belofsky, Nathan. *Strange Medicine*. New York, NY: Perigee Trade, 2013.

Bynum, William. *The History of Medicine*. New York, NY: Oxford University Press, 2008.

Hall, Tim. *History of Medicine*. New York, NY: Hachette Book Group, 2014.

Jackson, Mark. *The Oxford Handbook of the History of Medicine*. Oxford, England: Oxford University Press, 2013.

Kennedy, Michael T., M.D. *A Brief History of Disease, Science, and Medicine*. Irvine, CA: Asklepiad Press, 2009.

Lee, Thomas H. *Eugene Braunwald and the Rise of Modern Medicine*. Cambridge, MA: Harvard University Press, 2013.

Nuland, Sherwin B. *Doctors: The Illustrated History of Medical Pioneers*. New York, NY: Black Dog & Leventhal Publishers, 2008.

Parker, Steve. *Kill or Cure: An Illustrated History of Medicine*. London, England: DK, 2013.

Pickover, Clifford. *The Medical Book*. New York, NY: Sterling, 2012.

Rogers, Kara. *Medicine and Healers Through History*. New York, NY: Rosen Educational Services, 2011.

Rutkow, Ira. *Seeking the Cure: A History of Medicine in America*. New York, NY: Scribner, 2010.

Index

For main entries see contents page. References to medical figures are given only where mentioned other than their main entry.